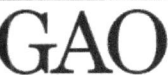

I0415856

July 2012

ANTHRAX

DHS Faces Challenges in Validating Methods for Sample Collection and Analysis

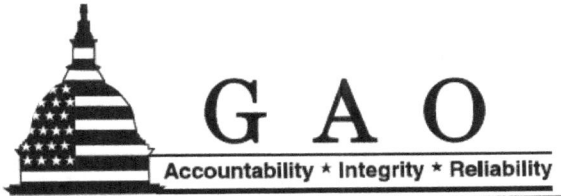

GAO
Accountability ★ Integrity ★ Reliability

GAO-12-488

ANTHRAX

DHS Faces Challenges in Validating Methods for Sample Collection and Analysis

Highlights of GAO-12-488, a report to congressional requesters

Why GAO Did This Study

In 2005, assessing federal agencies' activities for detecting *Bacillus anthracis* in postal facilities, GAO reported that the test results of their sampling were largely negative. GAO found that the agencies had not used validated sampling methods and approaches that would have given a defined level of confidence for negative results. Consequently, GAO recommended several actions. In this study, GAO was asked to identify the extent to which (1) DHS's actions have addressed GAO's recommendations regarding sampling, (2) the environmental sampling methods for *B. anthracis* spore detection in initial public health sampling and microbial forensic investigations have been validated, and (3) any challenges remain to completing validation. GAO analyzed agency documents and interviewed agency officials.

What GAO Recommends

To ensure validated sampling methods and approaches are available for decision makers to respond to an indoor *Bacillus anthracis* release, DHS should (1) update the strategic plan and its roadmap with an agreed scope and timelines, and (2) complete the validation project. The Secretary of HHS and the Administrator of EPA should support DHS's goal of achieving validated sampling methods and a statistically based sampling approach. DHS agreed with our recommendations; EPA and HHS disagreed with our recommendation to them, stating that such an approach was not feasible or necessary. We continue to believe a validated statistical sampling approach will provide a broader range of options for decision makers responding to future incidents.

View GAO-12-488. For more information, contact Timothy M. Persons, Chief Scientist, at (202) 512-6412 or personst@gao.gov.

What GAO Found

A workgroup—led by the U.S. Department of Homeland Security (DHS) and made up of DHS and the Centers for Disease Control and Prevention (CDC), the Environmental Protection Agency (EPA), the Federal Bureau of Investigation (FBI), and the National Institute of Standards and Technology (NIST)—has attempted to address GAO's recommendations to (1) validate environmental sampling methods for detecting *Bacillus anthracis* and (2) conduct studies to develop probability-based sampling approaches for indoor environments. This workgroup has taken some actions to validate environmental sampling methods (collection, transportation, preparation, analysis) and develop statistically based sampling approaches that will provide confidence statements when test results are negative. These activities were projected to be completed by fiscal year 2013, but delays are now expected.

While progress has been made in validating sampling methods for detecting *Bacillus anthracis* spores in indoor environments, their validation is not yet complete. Some studies have not begun. Although more is known about the methods' performance characteristics—such as their limits of detection—other aspects of the methods are unknown, such as false negative rates. CDC has validated the preparation and analysis but not the collection methods for the swab and wipe. CDC states that field validation would be too difficult and laboratory validation of collection methods is not required. However, experts GAO talked to stated that collection methods could be validated in a laboratory.

Agencies that perform environmental sampling take the lead in validating the sampling methods. The FBI does not typically use CDC's environmental sampling methods and validating its methods is outside the scope of the DHS-led workgroup. The FBI's environmental sampling methods are not validated but the agency relies on DHS's National Bioforensic Analysis Center (NBFAC) to validate its microbial forensic analytical methods. Thus, the FBI, through NBFAC, and CDC are attempting to validate analytical methods for *Bacillus anthracis* but neither is validating the collection methods. Nevertheless, improvements in sample collection procedures for the swab and wipe could be useful to the FBI in developing its sampling plans or in evaluating its sampling methods.

The workgroup must address several remaining challenges before the validation project can be completed: (1) clarifying the strategic plan's scope—some agencies believe it is overly ambitious and differ on whether it includes linking sampling results to a risk-based decision process—and determining whether the workgroup is to continue; (2) reaching consensus on the range of sampling approaches that should be available to decision makers in different phases of a response; (3) establishing realistic estimates of the time for completing prioritized validation activities; (4) addressing scientific gaps, such as assessing risk in the absence of dose-response data; and (5) ensuring the availability of funds for critical tasks. While validating the methods provides information on performance characteristics, human health risks from any particular level of exposure remain uncertain. Since the workgroup has invested about $12 million and considerable resources over about 7 years, it would be prudent for it to complete prioritized tasks. Thus, the workgroup may wish to consider carefully what work is needed and think strategically in terms of its investments and their potential benefits.

_____ United States Government Accountability Office

Contents

Tables

Figures

Abbreviations

CDC	Centers for Disease Control and Prevention
CFU	Colony forming unit
DFA	direct fluorescent antibody
DHS	U.S. Department of Homeland Security
DNA	deoxyribonucleic acid
DOD	U.S. Department of Defense
DOE	U.S. Department of Energy
EPA	Environmental Protection Agency
FBI	Federal Bureau of Investigation
HEPA	high-efficiency particulate air
HHS	U.S. Department of Health and Human Services
HSPD	Homeland Security Presidential Directive
IEC	International Electrotechnical Commission
INL	Idaho National Laboratory
ISO	International Organization for Standardization
LLNL	Lawrence Livermore National Laboratory
LRN	Laboratory Response Network
NBACC	National Biodefense Analysis and Countermeasures Center
NBFAC	National Bioforensic Analysis Center
NIOSH	National Institute for Occupational Safety and Health
NIST	National Institute of Standards and Technology
NRF	National Response Framework
PCR	polymerase chain reaction
PNNL	Pacific Northwest National Laboratory
SNL	Sandia National Laboratories
VSP	Visual Sample Plan
VSPWG	Validated Sampling Plan Working Group

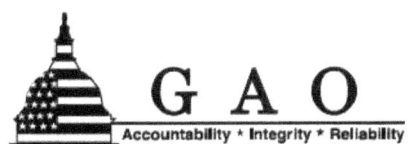

United States Government Accountability Office
Washington, DC 20548

July 31, 2012

The Honorable Fred Upton
Chairman
The Honorable Henry Waxman
Ranking Member
Committee on Energy and Commerce
House of Representatives

The Honorable Cliff Stearns
Chairman, Subcommittee on Oversight
  and Investigations
Committee on Energy and Commerce
House of Representatives

The Honorable Rush Holt
House of Representatives

Despite the fact that the bioterrorist use of *Bacillus anthracis* in 2001 highlighted federal agencies' poor preparation to respond to its intentional release, proposed refinements to the select agent list are not likely to affect *B. anthracis*—the bacteria that cause anthrax—as one of the nation's top biological threat agents.[1] The letters containing *B. anthracis* spores mailed in 2001 to members of the Congress and the media contaminated numerous federal and civilian facilities. Other mail routed

---

[1]Select agents are biological agents and toxins (1) that have the potential to pose a severe threat to public health and safety, to animal or plant health, or to animal or plant products and (2) whose possession, use, and transfer are regulated by select agent rules (7 C.F.R. Part 331, 9 C.F.R. Part 121, and 42 C.F.R. Part 73). The Centers for Control and Prevention (CDC) and U.S. Department of Agriculture (USDA) maintain a list of select agents and toxins (see www.selectagents.gov/Select%20Agents%20and%20Toxins%20Exclusions.html). The President's July 2010 Executive Order 13546 created a Federal Experts Security Advisory Panel, that was tasked with assisting the Secretaries of Health and Human Services (HHS) and Agriculture to determine risk-based tiers for the Select Agent List. The November 2010 report of the Advisory Panel, *Recommendations Concerning the Select Agent Program*, recommended that *B. anthracis* be listed as a Tier 1 agent. Tier 1 agents present the greatest risk of deliberate misuse with the most significant potential for mass casualties or devastating effects to the economy, critical infrastructure, or public confidence. HHS's and Agriculture's proposed rules, published in October 2011, would amend the Select Agent Regulations to include *B. anthracis* as a Tier 1 overlap select agent. See 76 Fed. Reg. 61,206 (Oct. 3, 2011); 76 Fed. Reg. 61,228 (Oct. 3, 2011).

GAO-12-488 Anthrax Detection

through these and other facilities in the postal network also became contaminated. Federal facilities in the Washington, D.C., area—including the U.S. Supreme Court, Walter Reed Army Institute of Research, the U.S. Department of Health and Human Services (HHS), and main State Department buildings—were later found to be contaminated.

Several federal agencies responded to that intentional release of *B. anthracis* spores in keeping with their respective roles. The Centers for Disease Control and Prevention (CDC) has a lead role in identifying agents and protecting the public's health, the Federal Bureau of Investigation (FBI) leads criminal investigations, and the Environmental Protection Agency (EPA) has the lead role in characterizing the extent and degree of contamination in the environment and in advising on decontamination. In 2005, we assessed and described federal agencies' activities to detect *B. anthracis* spores in the postal facilities, and the results of their testing, and we also examined the status of validation of the agencies' environmental detection activities.[2]

We reported in 2005 that when the contamination level in a building is extremely high and dispersed, the sampling approach and sampling methods may not be as critical if the purpose is to detect the presence of spores. In that report, we identified and focused on a contrasting scenario that was based on the 2001 *B. anthracis* attack—low-level contamination inside a building.[3]

In 2001, the sensitivity and specificity of the sampling methods that were used were not known—that is, how effective these methods were with regard to the number of *B. anthracis* spores they could detect—because

---

[2]GAO, *Anthrax Detection: Agencies Need to Validate Sampling Activities in Order to Increase Confidence in Negative Results*, GAO-05-251 (Washington, D.C.: March 31, 2005).

[3]In this report, we use sampling approach to refer to the selection of the locations of the sample areas from which material is collected (whether using probability sampling, other judgmental selection approaches, or some hybrid of those approaches to determine the specific sites for collection), as well as the determination of the number of such areas for collection. We use sampling methods to refer to four major steps necessary to quantify the material collected at the sample locations: implementing (1) a collection method (using devices such as a swab, swipe, or vacuum), and (2) a transportation method for storing and moving the collection devices to laboratories, (3) a preparation method for extracting material from the collection devices for analysis, and (4) conducting the analytic methods(s) for quantifying or classifying the extracted material. The sampling plan comprises the sampling approach and the sampling methods taken together.

these methods were not validated. Also, the agencies did not use probability sampling in their sampling approaches. Probability sampling makes it possible to estimate the confidence one has in the results of the sampling approach—even when all testing results are negative.[4] In simple terms, one can say whether it is likely that low-level contamination could have been missed only by chance even if all testing results are negative.

Because agencies did not use validated sampling methods or probability sampling, which would have allowed confidence statements about the estimates of contamination, we concluded that little could be said about the confidence that could be placed in the negative results generated from the agencies' initial testing—a concern under the scenario we have described.[5]

As a result, we recommended that the Secretary of Homeland Security ensure the validation of the sampling methods (collection, transport, extraction, or preparation, and analysis) so that performance characteristics, including limitations, are clearly understood and results can be correctly interpreted.[6] We also recommended that the Secretary see that appropriate investments are made in studies to develop probability-based sampling approaches that take into account the complexities of indoor environments (different surface materials and

---

[4]A probability sample, taken from a population (a collection of units or areas to be studied) is defined by the use of some randomization method that gives each unit in the population a known, nonzero probability of being selected and that uses those probabilities in a valid method of statistical analysis of the measurements. A probability sample allows for estimating levels of confidence about the estimates made. We use the term "negative" to indicate that a test result did not detect B. anthracis. HHS uses the term "non-detect" to describe that result, rather than "negative." When a test fails to detect B. anthracis because it is below the limit of detection of the method, then by our definition that test result is negative. A negative analytical result does not mean that B anthracis is absent or that the sampled area is free of contamination. Indeed it could be present below the limit of detection.

[5]By initial sampling, we refer to CDC's objectives for environmental sampling: rapid determination of the presence of B. anthracis spores.

[6]The process of sampling involves the sample collection method using a specific device, and storage and transporting collected samples to a laboratory, where they will be prepared for analysis. Evaluating each of these steps (and each method) in studies will determine their sensitivity, specificity, and other key performance characteristics, and is thus a key step in validating a method.

building architecture) so as to allow statements about the likelihood of contamination when results are negative as in the scenario we described.

In response, the U.S. Department of Homeland Security (DHS) agreed to take the lead in implementing our recommendations. In this context, you asked us to identify

1. the extent to which DHS's actions have addressed our recommendations,

2. the extent to which the environmental sampling methods for *B. anthracis* spore detection in initial public health sampling and microbial forensic investigations have been validated, and

3. any challenges to completing validation.

To do this, we reviewed and analyzed the relevant agencies' documentation of their validation efforts for the sampling methods they used to detect *B. anthracis* spores in indoor environments, with a focus primarily on those used during crisis management, the first phase of a response. We identified DHS's actions responding to the recommendations in our 2005 report regarding the sampling methods used for public health purposes, as well as its coordination of the interagency activities, by reviewing and analyzing pertinent documentation, including the 2006 interagency memorandum of understanding between CDC, DHS, EPA, and NIST; the 2007 interagency strategic plan and its periodically updated roadmaps; guidance documents, external review panel assessments, and independent assessments of building experiments; published validation studies; and funding data for and the management of the validation project, among others.

To determine the extent to which the environmental sampling methods applied in public health and microbial forensic investigations for detecting *B. anthracis* spores during initial sampling have been validated, we reviewed the definition of validation the DHS-led interagency workgroup—known as the Validated Sampling Plan Working Group (VSPWG)—adopted to guide its validation of the sampling methods. We assessed the extent to which DHS and the VSPWG have completed the activities in the validation project, including their progress in validating the sampling methods and evaluating sampling approaches, compared to the activities listed in the strategic plan's roadmap. We did not independently verify the validation data the agencies collected. We interviewed officials from within HHS, including CDC and its National Institute of Occupational Safety and Health (NIOSH), and the National Center for Emerging and Zoonotic Infectious Diseases; DHS; the Department of Defense (DOD); EPA; the FBI; and the National Institute of Standards and Technology (NIST) regarding the validation of sampling methods and the evaluation of sampling approaches. We visited the Department of Energy's (DOE) Pacific Northwest National Laboratory (PNNL) to obtain further information on some of its validation activities in the roadmap, such as its development and internal validation of pertinent sampling design modules in the Visual Sample Plan (VSP) software.

Further, we analyzed documentation that DHS, the FBI, and the National Bioforensic Analysis Center (NBFAC) provided us as well as other pertinent documentation, such as studies and reports on the methods and approaches the federal agencies, including the FBI, used for sampling facilities in the 2001 *B. anthracis* attack. We interviewed officials regarding microbial forensic methods within DHS, DOD, EPA, and NIST; we visited PNNL; and we interviewed and visited NBFAC and the FBI Laboratory at Quantico, Virginia.

We identified challenges that VSPWG has encountered in its validation efforts. We reviewed relevant DHS, FBI, VSPWG, and other related documentation. We discussed challenges to validating methods with officials from CDC, DHS, DOD, EPA, the FBI, NIOSH, and NIST. Finally, we asked scientists who had expertise in public health investigations to review and comment on a draft of our report. (Further details on our scope and methodology are in appendix I.)

We conducted our work from March 2010 through June 2012 in accordance with generally accepted government auditing standards. Those standards require that we plan and perform the audit to obtain sufficient, appropriate evidence to provide a reasonable basis for our findings and conclusions based on our audit objectives. We believe that the evidence we obtained provides a reasonable basis for our findings and conclusions based on our audit objectives.

Background

B. anthracis

Anthrax is an acute infectious disease caused by the spore-forming bacterium B. anthracis. It can infect humans but is most common in other warm-blooded animals such as herbivores. An intentional release of B. anthracis spores in October 2001 resulted in the death of five persons from inhalation anthrax. The most recent reported case of inhalation anthrax in the United States before October 2001 was in 1976. Since 2001, several cases of anthrax have resulted from natural occurrences—not bioterrorism.[7]

Under normal circumstances, human infection results from an occupational exposure to infected animals or animal products. For example, workers may be exposed to dead animals infected with anthrax or contaminated products such as wool, hides, or hair products. Human infection from natural causes is rare in the United States. Anthrax is not considered to be contagious, although there have been rare anecdotal reports that infection has been transmitted following contact with cutaneous lesions. Humans are infected (1) cutaneously, usually through a cut or an abrasion in the skin; (2) gastrointestinally, by ingesting food or drink that is contaminated with spores; and (3) by inhalation, by breathing B. anthracis spores into the lungs. Symptoms depend on how the disease is contracted but usually appear within 7 days. If recognized in time, the disease can be treated with appropriate antimicrobials.

---

[7]In 2006, in New York a man who had worked with African animal hides to make drums died from inhalation anthrax. In 2007, two people in Connecticut were treated for cutaneous anthrax traced to animal hides used to make African drums. In 2009, in New Hampshire a woman with gastrointestinal anthrax had attended a drumming session in which drums had been made from African animal hides. It was theorized that she had swallowed aerosolized spores. See CDC, "Gastrointestinal Anthrax after an Animal-Hide Drumming Event—New Hampshire and Massachusetts, 2009," *MMWR* 59 (28) 2010: 872-77; CDC, "Cutaneous Anthrax Associated with Drum Making Using Goat Hides from West Africa—Connecticut, 2007," *MMWR* 57 (23) 2008: 628-31; CDC, "Inhalation Anthrax Associated with Dried Animal Hides—Pennsylvania and New York City, 2006," *MMWR* 55 (2006): 280-82.

Agencies' Roles in Responding to a Biological Release Are Interrelated

The interrelated roles of the many federal agencies in planning for, responding to, and recovering from biological incidents are illustrated in figure 1.[8] DHS coordinates the federal government's overall response to or recovery from terrorist attacks, major disasters, or other emergencies.[9] CDC within HHS is the primary agency for the public health response to a biological terrorism attack or naturally occurring outbreak. Initial sampling of contaminated areas and treating exposed individuals may occur by other agencies before CDC's involvement (for example, a white powder incident). EPA is the primary agency for determining the extent and level of contamination in a biological terrorism attack or natural outbreak, which includes sampling for site characterization purposes.[10] It is also the primary agency for determining the plan for decontaminating contaminated areas. The FBI within the U.S. Department of Justice is the primary agency for the criminal investigation of incidents of bioterrorism.[11]

---

[8]Homeland Security Presidential Directive (HSPD) 5 describes the management of domestic incidents and directs the Secretary of DHS to develop a National Response Plan (now called the National Response Framework (NRF)), and HSPD-10 describes for the strategies for preventing, protecting against, and mitigating biological weapons attacks.

[9]The Homeland Security Act of 2002 made the Secretary of DHS responsible for coordinating the use of federal government resources when responding to or recovering from terrorist attacks, major disasters, or other emergencies under certain event conditions.

[10]HHS serves as the federal government's primary agency for the public health response to a biological terrorism attack or natural outbreak. In addition, HHS collaborates with the EPA in developing sampling strategies and sharing results when there is potential for environmental contamination. HHS also coordinates federal assistance to supplement state, tribal, and local resources in response to a public health and medical emergency. See NRF Biological Incident Annex. HSPD-10 notes that the EPA Administrator is developing, in coordination with other agencies, specific standards, protocols, and capabilities to address the risks of contamination following a biological weapons attack and developing strategies, guidelines, and plans for decontaminating persons, equipment, and facilities.

[11]According to HSPD-5, the attorney general has lead responsibility for criminal investigations of terrorist acts or terrorist threats made by individuals or groups inside the United States or directed at U.S. citizens or institutions abroad, where such acts are within the federal criminal jurisdiction of the United States. The criminal investigation of biological incidents or bioterrorism is under the purview of Justice, and DHS is designated to coordinate the overall response and recovery activities.

GAO-12-488 Anthrax Detection

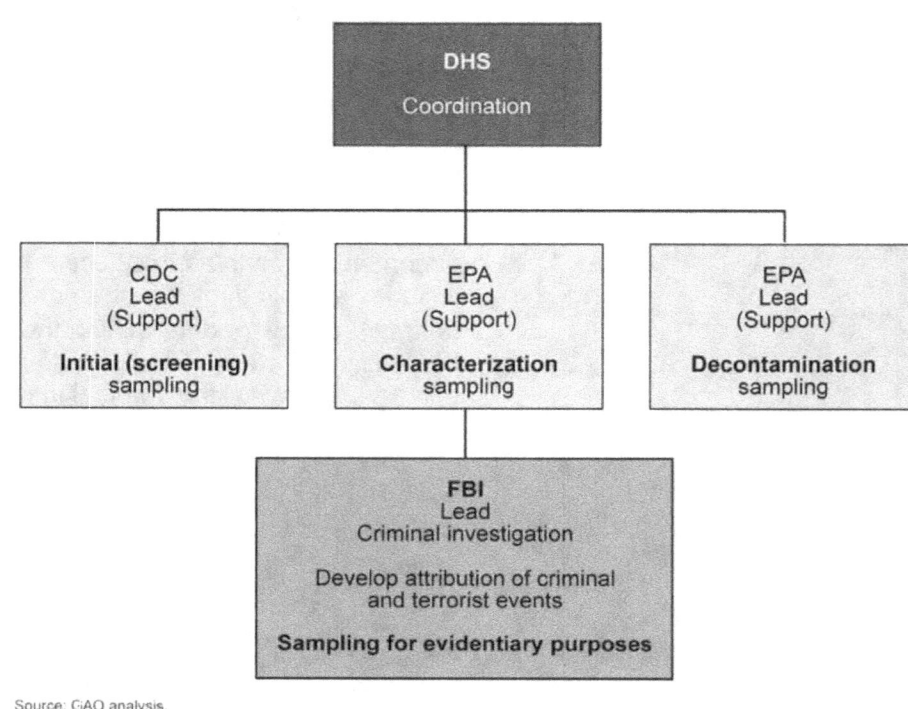

Source: GAO analysis.

Following a notification that *B. anthracis* has been released, the FBI would lead an investigation. Relevant agency partners, such as CDC and EPA, would also become involved. However, response roles and the order of notification (that is, which agencies are involved first) are variable, depending on the scenario (for example, the initial detection). For example, according to CDC, the Laboratory Response Network (LRN) and CDC work closely with the FBI (founding members of LRN) and hence analytical methods that will be used by public health for identifying and characterizing the agent may also be used by the FBI for attribution purposes.[12] Thus, while CDC and EPA are lead agencies for initial sampling and for site characterization and decontamination sampling, respectively, they would support an incident's criminal investigation—including a microbial forensics investigation—while DHS would coordinate it.

Crisis and Consequence Management

Crisis and consequence management are the two phases of response to a chemical, biological, or radiological incident. Crisis management may be managed by public health agencies and local, state, and federal law enforcement, which includes first responders.[13] During this phase, the FBI conducts a threat assessment that may include relevant agency partners. If it is determined that a biological threat agent has been released, an Incident Commander is designated and an incident command system is established. CDC and local, county, and state health agencies may also manage the public health consequences of an incident.

Sampling is conducted for different objectives throughout crisis management and consequence management. Public health sampling of a facility during crisis management involves initial sampling, in which environmental samples are collected to determine (through laboratory analysis) the agent type, relative concentration, and viability (see table 1). (Appendix II lists select agents and toxins.) According to CDC, initial sampling is most often conducted by a variety of local response agencies. Microbial susceptibility testing is also an important component of public health sampling as it informs treatment and post-exposure prophylaxis options.

---

[12]The LRN was established in 1999 to coordinate clinical diagnostic testing for bioterrorism. Its primary purpose on the biological side was to detect bio-threat agents within a number of specimen and sample types, especially since CDC was working closely with the FBI on preparedness and response needs for law enforcement. The LRN and its partners are to maintain an integrated national and international network of laboratories—currently more than 150—that are fully equipped to respond quickly to acts of chemical or biological terrorism, emerging infectious diseases, and other public health threats and emergencies. State and local public health laboratories are the bulk of these laboratories. They are qualified by CDC to analyze samples containing *B. anthracis* and other biological pathogens.

[13]Local fire officials or police officers or both are sent to the scene of reported hazards. A hazardous materials (HAZMAT) responder is a trained and certified individual who is a member of a hazardous material response team or who is qualified to respond to incidents involving toxic industrial chemicals or chemical warfare agents and other weapons of mass destruction or both.

Table 1: The Two Management Phases of a Response to a Biological Release

Crisis management		Consequence management		
Notification	**First response**	**Characterization**	**Decontamination**	**Clearance**
• A biological incident occurs at a suspect site • Agencies are notified	• HAZMAT, emergency, and public health actions are taken • Forensic investigation begins if credible threat • Initial environmental sampling and analysis at LRN laboratory to determine agent type, relative concentration, viability • Risk is communicated on the basis of the initial assessment of exposure risk, among other things	• A biological agent is characterized • Environmental sampling and analysis gather information about the contamination • Risk is assessed • Clearance goals are set	Equipment and facilities are decontaminated[a] Verification of decontamination	Clearance sampling and analysis assess the success of decontamination

Source: Adapted from DHS and EPA, *Draft Planning Guidance for Recovery Following Biological Incidents* (Washington, D.C.: May 2009), fig. 3. p. 38.

[a]After removal of contaminated clothing, patients should be instructed (or assisted, if necessary) to immediately shower with soap and water, to include shampooing hair. Potentially harmful practices, such as bathing patients with bleach solutions, are unnecessary and should be avoided.

Analyzing samples begins with the LRN whose main roles in the 2001 *B. anthracis* scenario were first to detect the event and then identify and characterize the threat agent. Exposure risk would be determined by the epidemiologists investigating the incident. Evidence from a microbial forensic investigation must meet the scientific community's standards for evidence as well as a criminal court for legal admissibility.[14] The FBI may use laboratories other than its own for analysis of samples, including

[14]Under the Federal Rules of Evidence, Rule 702, an expert witness is considered qualified to testify if, among other things, the testimony is the product of reliable principles and methods. The 1993 Supreme Court case, Daubert v Merrell Dow Pharmaceuticals (509 U.S. 579), significantly changed the admissibility of scientific evidence for Federal trial courts, making trial judges responsible for acting as gatekeepers to exclude unreliable scientific expert testimony. The Daubert case listed factors for judges to use in assessing the reliability of scientific expert testimony, including (1) whether the expert's technique or theory can be or has been tested, (2) whether the technique or theory has been subject to peer review, (3) the known or potential rate of error of the technique or theory when applied, (4) the existence and maintenance of standards and controls, and (5) whether the technique or theory has been generally accepted by a relevant scientific community.

those of CDC and the NBFAC, depending on its sampling requirements and available resources and personnel at those laboratories. Supporting DHS civilian biodefense, the NBFAC is a unit of DHS's National Biodefense Analysis and Countermeasures Center's (NBACC) applied science and technology laboratory. The NBFAC was established 3 years after the 2001 *B. anthracis* attack, in 2004, with the mission of conducting and facilitating the technical forensic analysis and interpretation of materials recovered after a biological attack. The NBFAC analyzes evidence from biocrime or terrorist attacks to obtain a "biological fingerprint" that will be used by the FBI to identify perpetrators and determine the origin and method of attack. To do this, the NBFAC is developing forensic tools, methods, and strain repositories for pathogens of concern.

In contrast, sampling for site characterization, decontamination and clearance purposes is done during consequence management. Characterization sampling is to determine the extent of contamination after a biological release has been confirmed. Specifically, site characterization sampling is to assess the nature (identity and properties) and extent (location and quantity) of contamination of an area or items, and to provide information necessary to decide where, what and how to decontaminate.[15] Decontamination refers to inactivating or reducing a contaminant in or on buildings or other areas, by physical, chemical, or other methods to meet a cleanup goal. CDC and EPA state that at this time the goal for indoor environments is "no detectable, viable spores of *B. anthracis* following post-decontamination sampling."[16] After decontamination, clearance sampling is conducted to provide a basis for determining whether the cleanup goal has been met.

Sampling for *B. anthracis*

Sampling generally refers to a portion, piece, or segment that is representative of a whole.[17] In this report, we use "sampling plan" to mean determining locations (sampling approach) in indoor facilities and the associated activities and procedures (sampling methods) to collect ,

---

[15]See DHS and EPA, *Remediation Guidance for Major Airports after a Bioterrorist Attack* (Washington, D.C.: November 2008).

[16]See CDC and EPA, *Interim Clearance Strategy for Environments Contaminated with Bacillus anthracis* (Washington, D.C., February 2012).

[17]According to ISO 17025, sampling is taking a representative part of a substance, material, or product for testing or calibrating the whole.

transport and prepare material taken from those locations for analysis. Preparation involves extracting material from the collected samples, while analysis is those processes used in the laboratory to measure and quantify sampled material and identify and characterize a biological contaminant.

In deciding on a sampling plan, the analyst must consider such things as sampling or non-sampling error—for example, errors that occur when some locations are inaccessible for collecting a sample (see app. III for information on the role of sampling and nonsampling errors). Generally, environmental samples for a biological agent are primarily collected from inanimate surfaces and from the air but can also be collected from water and soil if needed. Samples are collected with a specific sample collection device (for example, a swab) while following specific procedures, methods, or protocols to determine whether a sample is positive or negative for the presence of a particular biological organism, such as *B. anthracis*.

Figure 2 illustrates the steps in the sampling method for *B. anthracis*, beginning with a particular collection device (for example, the swab), and ending with preparation and analysis of the collected samples.

Figure 2: Sampling Method: Sample Collection, Transportation, Preparation and Analysis

Sample collection	Sample transportation	Sample preparation	Sample analysis
1	**2**	**3**	**4**
From surfaces or air or both, using specified methods	From facility to laboratory, under appropriate conditions	At the laboratory using specified methods to extract spores from the sample media for analysis	Of living organisms in preliminary tests and confirmatory tests

Source: GAO analysis of CDC, EPA, and USPS data.

Note: Sample analysis may not require the presence of living organisms as in the case of material analyzed in polymerase chain reaction (PCR) directly without the prior growth of organisms.

The Sampling Method

Sample material from selected sample locations goes through the four steps depicted in figure 2. Material is collected by means of specific devices (such as a swab, wipe, surface vacuum, or air sampler) using specific collection procedures, and is then transported to a laboratory where associated protocols and procedures are used for measurement (such as preparation and analysis). Sample collection devices are of several types and material. Premoistened swabs are typically used to collect samples from small, nonporous surfaces such as within crevices, around corners, or on supply air diffusers, air return grills, and hard to reach places. Premoistened wipes or cellulose sponges (for example, sponge sticks) are typically used to collect samples from larger, nonporous surfaces. (See figure 3 for a swab and wipe). Vacuums may be used for sampling porous surfaces.

Figure 3: Cellulose Sponge Wipe and Macrofoam Swab

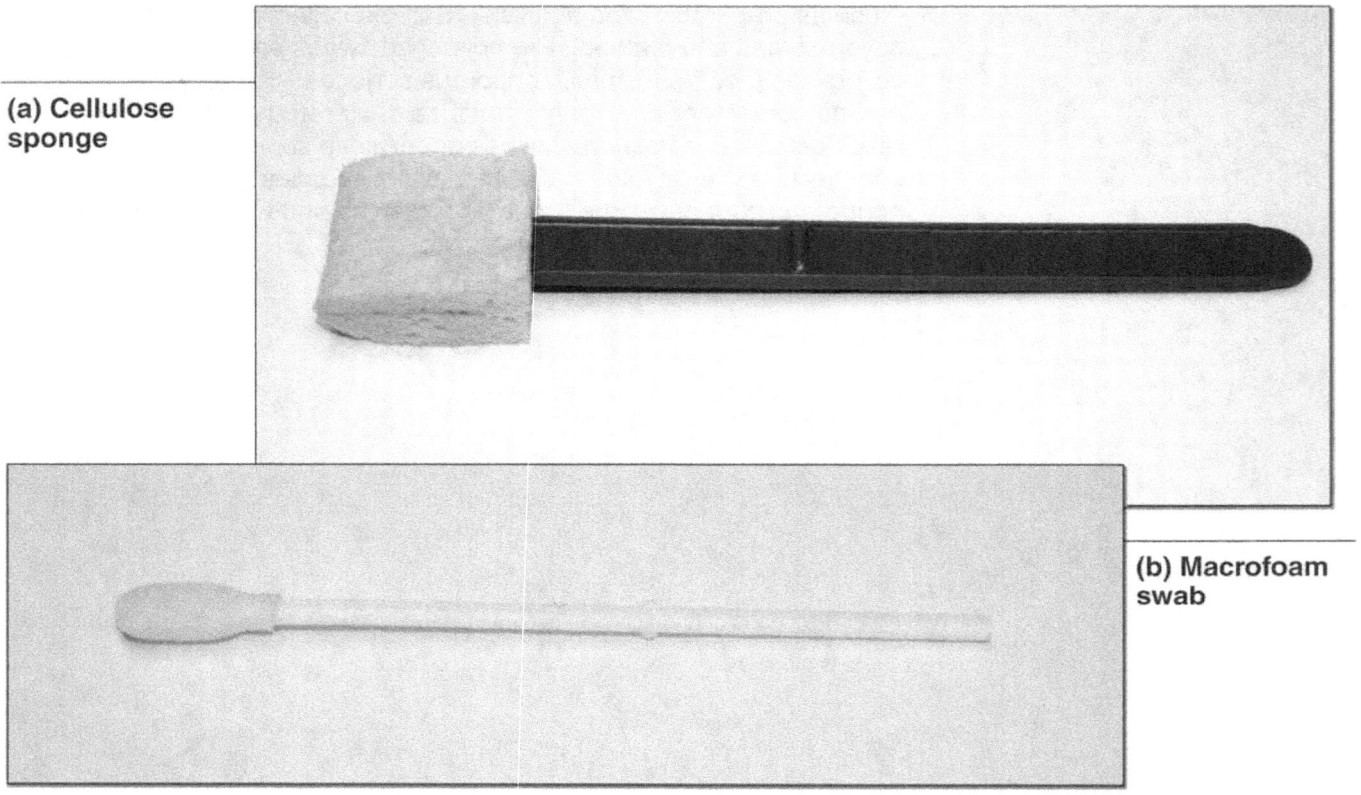

(a) Cellulose sponge

(b) Macrofoam swab

Source: CDC.

Note: (top) A 1-1/5 inch by 3 inch cellulose sponge is folded over a handle, such as the 3M™ Sponge-Stick. (bottom) A 3/16 inch thick medical-grade polyurethane foam head, 100 pores per inch, is thermally bonded to a polypropylene stick, such as the Sterile Foam Tipped Applicators Scored with Thumb Stop.

Collection devices are often used at a single location but they can also be used at more than one location. Such use is called a composite sample. Composite sampling results from sampling several locations (as opposed to only one location) with different sides of, for example a wipe, which then forms a new (composite) sample. Bulk samples may help detect the presence of contamination on entire, or parts of, building materials. Bulk samples may be challenging due to safety concerns (could cause secondary spreading of spores from contaminated samples) thus they should be used with caution. In addition, recovery of spores from these types of samples may be unpredictable thus interpreting the results may also be problematic. Also, air sampling using a variety of filters may be used to characterize the number of *B. anthracis* spores in the air.[18]

Preparation for and analysis of the collected samples will involve a variety of laboratory methods: LRN-validated processing methods are available to identify the specific agent (for example, bacteria or virus), the species and strain (for example, *B. anthracis* Ames), whether it is virulent or is antibiotic resistant (for example, by identifying the genetic materials that promote survival). Analytical methods for identifying *B. anthracis* may be microbiologic, such as culture, PCR, phage lysis, motility testing, for strain identification.[19]

VSPWG Has Taken Several Actions to Address GAO's Recommendations

In 2006, DHS's Science and Technology Directorate, in concert with other federal stakeholder agencies, established VSPWG, a management structure, under a 2006 interagency memorandum of understanding. CDC, EPA, the FBI, and NIST are VSPWG's principal members, according to DHS.[20] Led by DHS, VSPWG (1) implemented an interagency draft strategic plan in 2007 containing a roadmap of validation activities, (2) adopted an International Organization for Standardization (ISO) standard for validation of the sampling methods, and (3) supported the development of pertinent statistically-based

---

[18]A variety of filter media (gelatin, polytetrafluoroethylene, and the like) can be attached to pumps to collect air samples. Less frequently, impactors and liquid impingers can also be used to collect air samples where spores are collected on appropriate agar plates or in appropriate impinger liquid. Multistage impactors can be used to estimate spore size as well as air concentration.

[19]LRN-approved tests for detecting *B. anthracis* are at www.bt.cdc.gov/agent/anthrax/lab-testing/approvedlrntests.asp. PCR is a laboratory method in which a deoxyribonucleic acid (DNA) molecule is extracted from a sample and then analyzed with a specific procedure to detect the genetic code of known pathogens, such as anthrax. PCR can be used to diagnose disease by identifying genetic DNA material commonly found in all *B. anthracis* strains, among other things.

[20]DOD also played a role in some workgroup activities. Several laboratories of the U.S. Department of Energy (DOE) that are not VSPWG members, such as the Idaho National Laboratory (INL), PNNL, and Sandia National Laboratories (SNL), also assist in VSPWG's validation efforts. An external review panel is to advise VSPWG.

GAO-12-488 Anthrax Detection

sampling design modules in the VSP software, including a combined judgmental and random statistical sampling approach.[21]

Strategic Plan and Roadmap

The 2007 draft strategic plan focused on activities related only to environmental sampling in response to a biological incident involving *B. anthracis* spores in a facility. It addressed the full range of sampling and analytic activities related to the public health investigation, response to, and remediation of known contamination by *B. anthracis* spores disseminated as a powder or aerosol within a facility.

In the plan, the sampling methods that VSPWG was to validate for *B. anthracis* spores after a specific incident include the following:

1. sample collection from air and porous and nonporous surfaces, among others;

2. maintenance of sample integrity during transportation from a site of potential contamination (where samples were collected) to, and in storage at, the analytical laboratory;

3. preparation of samples: extracting spores from the samples at the laboratory for analysis; and

4. analysis in preliminary and confirmatory tests.

Also, the VSPWG planned to develop guidance for constructing scenario-specific sampling plans.

---

[21]In this report, statistically-based sampling encompasses any sampling with a statistical basis, including probabilistic and the combined judgmental and random sampling approach. The VSP is a software tool of many modules. For example, it has sampling design modules for soil, groundwater, sediments, surfaces, and unexploded ordnance site characterization. VSP's development has been supported by several federal agencies. The developer—PNNL—created modules containing sampling approaches that will allow confidence statements by a decision maker—that is, the VSP biological and chemical contamination modules. These modules include probability-based statistical sampling designs and the algorithms pertinent to within-building sampling that allow an investigator to prescribe or evaluate confidence levels of conclusion based on data collected as guided by the statistical sampling designs, according to PNNL. In this report, we refer only to pertinent modules in the VSP software, generally the combined judgmental and random sampling approach. For more information on the VSP software, see http://vsp.pnnl.gov/description.stm.

VSPWG's roadmap identifies, among other things, (1) time lines for validating sampling methods and completing other activities, (2) the lead agency responsible for each task in the roadmap, and (3) funding status (whether funded or unfunded). VSPWG revised the 2007 roadmap twice—most recently in August 2011. Completing all the validation activities in the 2011 roadmap is scheduled for the end of fiscal year 2013; however, delays are now anticipated because of budget constraints, according to DHS. Although DHS is responsible for tracking milestones in the roadmap, it has no leverage to ensure that milestones are addressed efficiently, according to a DHS official, because validation activities are generally funded by workgroup participant agencies within their own program prioritization schemes. Further, according to this official, prioritization of activities generally results from VSPWG consensus, with funding not necessarily correlated strongly with priority.

Activities in the roadmap with respect to sampling methods and approaches include, for example, (1) VSPWG's developing a draft "sampling strategy" guidance document for informing the development of sampling plans that meet decision makers' needs in a response; (2) evaluating sampling approaches, including the combined judgmental and random approach, (3) conducting exercises in a vacant INL building to evaluate the use of probability based sampling approaches using swab and wipe sampling methods, (4) validation of the sampling methods, and (5) examining uncertainties in sampling and addressing identified performance gaps through controlled chamber studies. According to DHS, the roadmap was a product of the consensus all participating agencies.

In 2007, DHS established an external review panel, through the Homeland Security Studies and Analysis Institute, of four subject matter experts to advise VSPWG and review its work.[22] DHS officials told us in March 2012 that it had decided to disband the original external review panel, primarily for its diminishing ability to maintain an independent perspective through its lengthy engagement with VSPWG. A new external

---

[22]In July 2011, DHS stated that the external review panel was to "review the objective data that was used to determine the inclusion of component processes (sample collection, sample transportation, sample preparation, and sample analysis), and through consideration of the validity of the component parts of the overall process and its execution, (1) provide an informed assessment of the validity of the process, and (2) assess the statistical validity of observed parameters associated with sampling methods."

review panel with different members is to be created. In September 2011, DHS informed us that a list of possible panelists had been drawn up, assessed by the institute, and sent to VSPWG members for their approval. As of March 2012, DHS stated that principal interagency stakeholders had not agreed on panel members, and DHS had not established this new panel.

The Scope VSPWG's Effort Needs Clarification

Some VSPWG officials told us on March 8, 2012, that the 2007 strategic plan was overly ambitious and unlikely to achieve its validation goals. According to DHS, the strategic plan reflects the original interagency scope but might be more comprehensive than VSPWG's scope can realistically accommodate because of the limitations of funding and technology. Whether its goals might not be met, DHS stated, is more a reflection of the realities of funding and technology and the commitment of VSPWG agencies to carry out their originally agreed upon tasks.

VSPWG members also disagree on whether the 2007 strategic plan includes risk assessment activity. Some VSPWG members believe that risk assessment is not part of method validation, being outside VSPWG's scope. DHS believes it is implicit. The intended purpose of the site-specific sampling plan—which will require the use of sampling methods and sampling approaches—is to inform a decision. Therefore, if the outcome of that sampling plan and the process used to develop it do not adequately inform a decision process, then the plan and supporting process will have failed. DHS stated that the external review panel also took this position in January 2010 when it concluded that VSPWG could not address GAO's recommendations without discussing risk assessment and risk management issues, although the panel did not provide guidance on how VSPWG could achieve them. One panelist initially questioned whether risk management was within VSPWG's charter.[23] According to DHS, the overall strategy and process for developing site-specific sampling plans will be validated in practice when an event in the scope of

---

[23]According to documentation we reviewed, the panel stated in a January 2010 teleconference that GAO's recommendations (within the charter of VSPWG) could not be addressed without discussing the risk assessment and risk management issues associated with making a clearance decision based on sampling data. In December 2009, the panel had raised the issue of risk management and acceptable risk, stating that it is through risk management that VSPWG should ultimately establish a link between sampling decisions and "no one gets sick." It was eventually agreed that VSPWG would combine risk management with risk assessment. The panel was to prepare a white paper to guide VSPWG.

the strategic plan occurs. However, practicing the process will only involve the execution of a sampling plan and a decision based on the result of using that plan. DHS stated that the notion of incorporating an exercise that considers both is in an update of the roadmap.[24] However, this exercise cannot be realistically done for a range of scenarios.

According to HHS, VSPWG was not tasked with evaluating risk assessment and it is not within VSPWG's scope. According to EPA, risk assessment is a separate scientific work area. It cannot be included in the validation of sampling and analysis methods. Validation helps establish the limit of detection for a method, which can ultimately provide a confidence in positive and negative results. Depending on the criteria used, risk assessment may provide risk estimates that relate to spore exposure concentrations number, which may either be well within or outside the limit of detection of the sampling and analyses methods.

In light of the above, further VSPWG clarification is needed on what is required to achieve process validation. While we understand that a risk assessment is needed in an agency's response to an incident, and that risk-based decisions will be supported by data from sampling, among other things, validating this additional process appears to be beyond the scope of the current strategic plan because it is not stated explicitly there. Consequently, this issue is open to differing interpretations. Identifying what needs to be done to complete the validation project requires VSPWG's consensus on the validation requirements, which is not due until the third quarter of fiscal year 2012, and further delays are expected.[25]

Activities in the 2011 roadmap related to completing validation include the following:

1. identifying requirements for process validation,

2. conducting independent validation,

---

[24]DHS did not identify this exercise, but the 2011 roadmap lists a task under "sampling strategy" for all VSPWG to "evaluate the need for additional field exercises."

[25]Commenting on a draft of this report, DHS stated that this milestone will be delayed by recent funding cuts affecting all principal participant agencies.

3. addressing identified deficiencies, and

4. conducting process validation.

VSPWG Adopted ISO 17025 for Validation

In 2005, we reported that most agency officials and scientists agreed that the sampling methods had not been validated but differed on the procedures necessary to validate them. Therefore, we recommended that the methods be validated—guided by an agreed-on definition of validation—so that their performance characteristics and limitations can be clearly understood and their results can be correctly interpreted. Validation, as it is generally understood, is a formal, empirical process in which the overall performance characteristics of a given method are determined and certified by an independent validating authority as (1) meeting the requirements for the intended application and (2) conforming to applicable standards. In 2007, VSPWG adopted the definition of validation of the sampling methods contained in ISO 17025, *General Requirements for the Competence of Testing and Calibration Laboratories,* which states that "Validation is the confirmation by examination and the provision of objective evidence that the particular requirements for a specific intended use are fulfilled."[26]

ISO 17025 focuses on the validation of laboratory methods, such as CDC's LRN-validated preparation and analysis methods for the swab and wipe, which we discuss later in this report.[27] It would also apply to the validation of EPA's rapid viability PCR method following EPA's Forum on

---

[26]ISO/IEC 17025:2005, *Technical Corrigendum* 1, Sec. 5.4.5, 2006-08-1 5. ISO 17025 is intended to facilitate cooperation between laboratories and others in exchanging information and experience and to assist in harmonizing standards and procedures. IEC is the International Electrotechnical Commission. The standard applies to all organizations performing tests or calibrations such as first-, second-, and third-party laboratories and laboratories where testing is part of inspection and product certification.

[27]The VSPWG roadmaps include validation of the CDC swab and wipe methods, developed through the LRN.

Environmental Measurement validation process.[28] ISO 17025 gives general guidance on what the validation of a method could include, such as evaluation of performance parameters in interlaboratory testing (objective evidence) and examination of a method's uncertainties to make sure it is fit for its intended use or application.[29] The standard notes that validation may include procedures for sampling, handling, and transportation but that testing deemed necessary to meet designated performance or other requirements is up to the user and the validating entity. ISO 17025 does not require independent validation.[30] VSPWG intended to use the ISO 17025 definition of validation to guide its validation of the activities described in the interagency memorandum of understanding.

In contrast, sampling components can be validated in a laboratory setting but concepts and guidance cannot. Components such as the collection methods, packaging and shipping protocols, preparation and analysis methods, and statistical analysis tools such as a statistical model's algorithms can be examined and validated. However, as previously discussed, DHS is also considering validation in terms of a broader process—one in which sampling data will support decisions within a risk-based framework. Therefore, these interlinked processes will have to be broken down into the component parts to determine what can and cannot be validated.

However, it is not yet clear how these processes will be validated in a manner that is consistent with ISO 17025. This issue will be resolved once VSPWG determines the requirements and validation criteria and

---

[28]EPA anticipates a logical path of multilaboratory validation of its rapid-viability PCR method with selected sample types and publication, depending on further research in fiscal years 2012-13 and the availability of required funding. Rapid-viability PCR is an analytic method of detecting live spores of *B. anthracis* Ames in environmental samples, including those from air filters, surface wipes, and water. Intended to shorten the time it takes to analyze a sample, it is to be used in a response to a potential indoor or outdoor wide-area *B. anthracis* attack. See also S. Létant and others, "Rapid-Viability PCR Method for Detection of Live, Virulent *Bacillus anthracis* in Environmental Samples," *Applied Environmental Microbiology* 77 (July 2011): 6570-78.

[29]See app. VIII for information on performance parameters.

[30]Laboratories must document their validation procedures and testing results, but publication is required only for methods that became international standards. Accreditation is considered a third-party attestation that an accredited laboratory has demonstrated its competence to carry out specific tests.

develops a validation plan and once an independent reviewer concludes that the validation criteria have been satisfied consistent with VSPWG's definition of validation, One way to facilitate this process would be to develop a validation master plan that specified the validation criteria (including method performance quantities to be estimated and, for each sampling method, a report indicating its completion of the validation criteria).[31]

VSPWG Supported the Development of a Statistically-Based Sampling Approach

We reported in 2005 that using a judgmental sampling approach and sampling methods that were not validated meant that no one could interpret negative results with statistical confidence. Our concern was for a specific scenario in the 2001 *B. anthracis* attack—that is, low-level *B. anthracis* spore contamination inside a building in which contamination could not be detected and no definitive statement about whether it was contaminated could be made with a degree of statistical confidence. We recommended that appropriate investments be made in studies to

---

[31]A validation master plan drives a structured approach to validation projects that will allow problems to be addressed before they become crises. A validation master plan is essentially a scope document that defines the critical systems to be validated and the appropriate approach and sequence in which to validate them. Its main objective is to outline, in sufficient detail, an approach to developing documented evidence that these critical systems consistently perform as designed and meet predetermined quality attributes. It should outline the type of activities to be performed and the sequence for performing them. For example, a validation master plan might include the objective, scope, approach, responsibilities, overall process description, processes to be validated, protocol requirements, general acceptance criteria, validation criteria, and involved personnel. For each sampling method, validation criteria might specify method performance quantities to be estimated and the uncertainties of the estimates quantified. A "validation report" could document the completion of the validation criteria.

develop probability-based sampling approaches that would take into account the complexities of indoor environments.[32]

VSPWG has supported development of a combined judgmental and random sampling approach, a statistical sampling approach as a module in the VSP software. This sampling approach, as well as others, is discussed in VSPWG's draft sampling strategy guidance—*Environmental Sampling Strategy for Bacillus anthracis during Crisis and Consequence Management.* VSPWG also conducted indoor experiments in a vacant INL building to evaluate the sampling approaches. Table 2 describes the status of these efforts.

[32]The need to understand the error characteristics of sampling approaches and sampling methods is emphasized by the early activities; there were largely negative results for 286 postal facilities. CDC officials stated in May 2012 that factors other than the lack of validated methods or sampling approaches might have contributed to these results. CDC also noted that no human cases of anthrax resulted from reoccupying the contaminated buildings after they were cleared through the environmental sampling completed at that time. For one facility—not expected to be contaminated—it took several sampling events to identify the contamination. Postal Service contractors used dry swabs to sample the facility twice—collecting 53 samples on November 11 and 64 samples on November 21—after a case of inhalation anthrax in a postal customer was confirmed. All test results for the contractors' sampling were negative. On November 25, CDC collected 60 remoistened swabs. Still, all results were negative. Finally, CDC performed "extensive and directed sampling" on November 28, using multiple methods—swabs, wet wipes, and HEPA vacuums. This time, of 202 samples, 4 wet wipes and 2 HEPA vacuum samples were positive. Some samples from the mail sorting machines were positive for *B. anthracis* spores, including a sample collected from a machine that primarily processed letter mail. The sample was found to contain about 3 million colony-forming units (CFU). But it took several sampling events to identify the spores in the mail processing equipment. While the sample from the machine containing 3 million CFUs was collected on November 28, 2001, another machine was sampled 5 times, and a total of 77 samples were collected, before *B. anthracis* spores were eventually found in an area that held mail for the ill postal customer. This particular machine would have sorted mail by the customer's carrier route and address. This facility is a good illustration of the complexities of sampling.

Table 2: VSPWG's Actions to Develop and Evaluate Sampling Approaches

Action	Completed	Ongoing	Additional information
Development activity			
Draft sampling strategy guidance document		✓	Includes sampling methods and approaches that could be employed in a response; annual updates are to include improved procedures
Develop and internally validate sampling design in VSP software		✓	PNNL developed a module in the VSP software that combined judgmental and random sampling. The sampling module can be used to develop site-specific sampling plans; its sampling algorithms were internally validated in 2009. The combined judgmental and random sampling approach is being improved and external validation is planned
Building exercises			
INL-1 in fiscal year 2007	✓		Conducted by DHS, DOD, EPA, and PNNL
INL-2 in fiscal year 2008	✓		DHS, DOD, and EPA evaluated various sampling approaches, including one that was probability based
Evaluate the need for additional field exercises		✓	All VSPWG member agencies planned an evaluation for the first half of fiscal year 2012

Source: GAO analysis.

August 2010 draft sampling strategy guidance provides information on various sampling methods such as swabs and wipes and on how to sample in a building so as to inform decision makers on response, decontamination, and reoccupancy. It also discusses various sampling approaches such as judgmental, probabilistic, combined judgmental and random, and composite sampling. The guidance is intended to inform the development of sampling plans that meet the needs of federal, state, local, and tribal decision makers when they are while making incident response, decontamination, and reoccupancy decisions when a release of *B. anthracis* has been detected. Following concern about the content of the guidance among some VSPWG agencies, it was eventually agreed that it should be a compendium of all available approaches and methods without preferring one approach over another. DHS states that it is now working with VSPWG to develop a consensus technical guidance document as originally planned under the memorandum of understanding.[33] We have not been provided a copy of the most recent

---

[33]The VSPWG memorandum of understanding defines a sampling strategy as a set of operating precepts and diagnostic tools (including sample collection methods, such as a swab; packaging and shipping protocols; recovery, preparation, and analytical methods such as culture; and statistical analysis packages) that are combined to confidently explain a specific hypothesis. In contrast, a sampling plan is a documented approach for field execution that captures the specific combination of operating precepts and diagnostic tools for a given site-specific scenario to explain a specific hypothesis.

version, but we understand that it is awaiting final review and approval for joint CDC, DHS, and EPA issuance.

Sampling Approaches Differ by Response Phase and Contamination Level

Indoor scenarios involving high-level and low-level contamination may use different sampling approaches. An appropriate sampling plan considers the phase of an incident response (for example, initial assessment, site characterization, and clearance) and uses of judgmental sampling, statistical sampling, and combinations of these. A heavily contaminated building in which initial sampling results using judgmental sampling provided some positive results would not need statistical sampling because it would be known that contamination was present. In contrast, in areas of suspected low-level or no contamination, a decision maker might want to make a statistical confidence statement, particularly if a risk assessment indicated that contamination was likely even though initial sample results were negative and vulnerable individuals could have been exposed. Table 3 lists some advantages and disadvantages of the two sampling approaches.

Table 3: Some Advantages and Disadvantages of Judgmental and Probability-based Sampling Approaches

Approach	Judgmental	Probability-based
Advantage	• Efficient approach with site knowledge • Easy to implement • May require fewer samples than in probabilistic sampling • Results support general inferences about the likelihood of contamination	• Allows quantification of confidence associated with estimates • Allows statistical inferences • Can handle decision error criteria • Can supplement results from judgmental sampling for greater combined confidence • Enables decision makers to designate a confidence level
Disadvantage	• Since results do not support statistical inferences; judgmental sampling can have no confidence levels • Depends on expert knowledge to identify sampling locations • Relies heavily on conceptual site model accuracy • Depends on subjective judgment to interpret data relative to sampling objectives	• May be difficult to identify random locations • May require more time and expense • Is likely to require more samples than judgmental sampling, depending on decision maker's required confidence level for the probability sample

Source: Adapted from EPA, *Guidance on Choosing a Sampling Design for Environmental Data Collection for Use in Developing a Quality Assurance Project Plan*, EPA QA/G-5S (Washington, D.C.: December 2002). .

VSPWG Supported Development of Combined Judgmental and Random Sampling

With funding from CDC, DHS, and EPA, NIOSH and PNNL jointly developed a statistically-based sampling approach that combines judgmental and probabilistic sampling for site characterization or clearance purposes. The combined judgmental and random sampling algorithm can be used to determine the required number and location of probability-based (random or systematic) samples—given the planned or actual number of judgmental samples—to provide a specified confidence that a specified level of contamination is not exceeded, including very low levels. Thus, the number of samples to be collected can be controlled by the level of confidence that users, or decision makers, require for the use of the sampling results.

Probability-based Sampling Is Likely to Be at Decision Makers' Discretion

The determination of what constitutes an acceptable level of confidence when using statistical sampling approaches is most likely to be based on a number of factors, paramount being the perceived risk to human health. In addition, statistical sampling plans are designed to optimize their ability to detect spores with as few samples as possible. According to EPA, since confidence levels in its experience need to be between 90 percent and 100 percent to be acceptable, thousands of samples are needed for a single building. EPA states that laboratory capacity is not enough to support the analysis of the number of samples that would be generated by probability-based sampling.

We agree that when taking a simplistic approach to sampling—if the contaminant were, on average, on fewer than 1 in 250 possible samples, throughout all possible samples—would indeed require about 1000 samples or more because the probability of detection decreases as the contaminant becomes more scarce. But professional samplers are expected to work with agencies and others with substantive knowledge to better understand how the contaminant was released and how it might have spread through a building. Doing so would allow the sampler to devise sampling approaches, including site-specific sampling plans that would create sampling units with a much higher probability of detecting the contaminant and, thus, a lower sample size. Consequently, costs would be lower and strain on laboratory resources would be less.

Decisions on the need for additional sampling—after initial sampling has been conducted—will depend in the future on the decision makers' needs. Such decisions will be based in part on the results of a risk assessment—along with consultations with others, such as subject matter experts—regarding the likelihood of contamination. This could be particularly important where initial sampling results are negative. However, risk-related information, such as dose-response relationships, is lacking, preventing experts from estimating the risk of exposure and subsequent risk of disease.

Therefore, the confidence level—that a decision maker determines is acceptable when statistical sampling is conducted—may ultimately mean any level that presents more risk than a decision maker is willing to take. That may well be an economic decision influenced by the cost of quantifying such levels relative to the expected cost of not doing so.

As shown in figure 4, the decision to use probability-based sampling would be at the discretion of the decision maker, such as an Incident commander who is heading an incident command in a bioterrorism incident.

Figure 4: Level of Contamination and Initial Sampling Approach

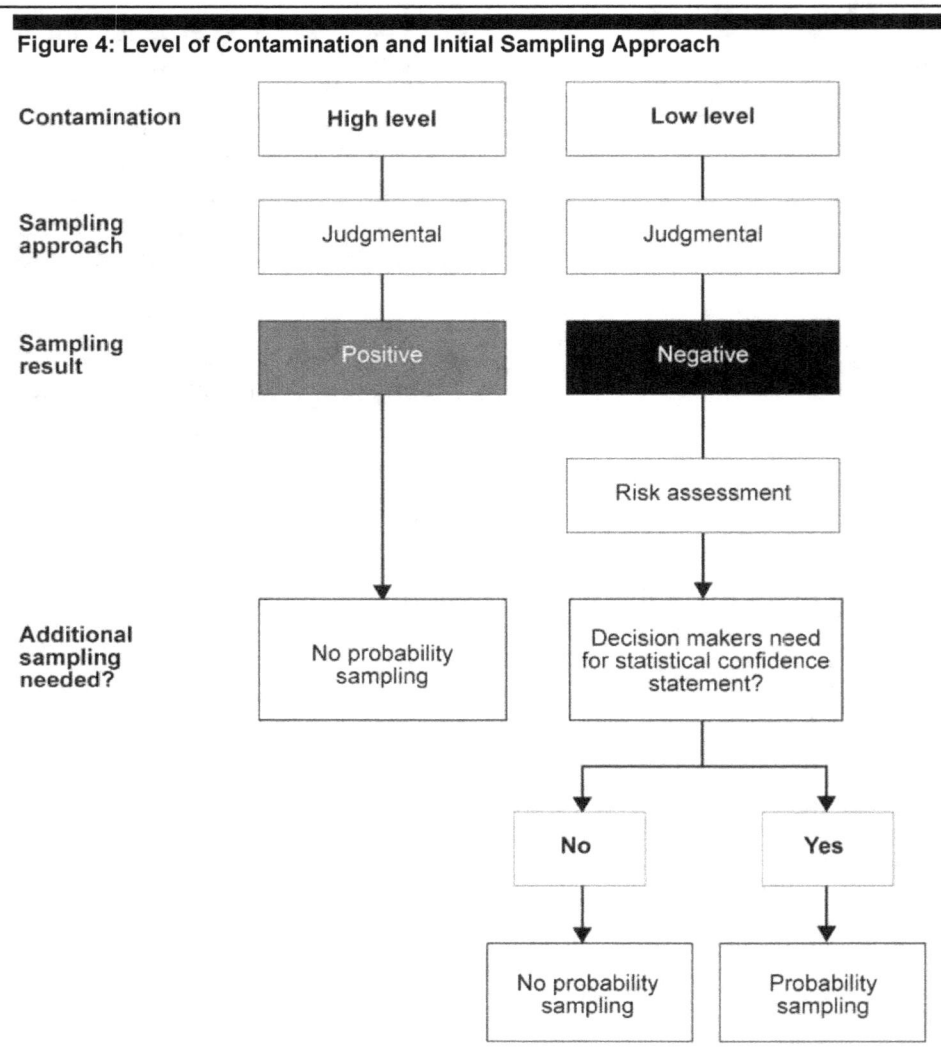

Source: GAO analysis.

Combined Judgmental and Random Sampling Generates a Confidence Statement When Results Are Negative

The combined judgmental and random sampling approach involves first identifying scenario-specific variables, decision-rule options, and statistical and modeling problems associated with sampling for B.

anthracis spores and then generating a confidence statement when sampling results are negative.[34] The Bayesian approach underlying combined judgmental and random sampling incorporates what is known about the chances that judgment samples were contaminated, thus supplementing judgmental approaches and allowing statistical inferences about the likelihood that contamination is present.[35] It can be used to determine the required number and location of probabilistic (random or systematic) samples, given the planned number of judgmental samples.

PNNL internally validated the VSP software algorithms in 2009, including the combined judgmental and random sampling design, reporting that the validation effort focused on four VSP sampling designs based on several sampling objectives that were considered pertinent for sampling within a building after a biological attack.[36] Validating each VSP sampling design involved applying each design to a simulated site (in some cases, different areas of the site), taking the number of samples suggested by the VSP to meet the design parameters, and using the VSP's decision rules to conclude whether or not the total decision unit was contaminated. To validate that the sampling designs could meet a 95-percent confidence requirement, samples were repeatedly taken, and the results used, in over 10,000 trials; for each trial, the result determined whether the site could be declared contaminated. The results from the simulations validated the selected VSP sampling designs. PNNL reported that the algorithms within VSP that calculated sample size, sample location, and the conclusions from statistical tests provided the information expected

---

[34]Results can be negative if (1) samples were not collected from places where *B. anthracis* was present, (2) the detection limit of the sampling method was greater than the contamination level, (3) not enough samples were collected, (4) not enough spores were recovered from the sample material, (5) analysis of the sample extract did not detect *B. anthracis* spores, or (6) *B. anthracis* was not present. According to HHS, sources of error can be varied and also can include whether culture or PCR was being used to detect the presence of *B. anthracis*. Assuming clearance sampling, then residual decontaminant could be present, which inhibits the growth of the organism; or, it could be an error.

[35]Bayesian probability is an interpretation of the concept of probability, belonging to the category of evidential probabilities. Bayesian interpretation of probability is an extension of logic that enables reasoning with uncertain statements. To evaluate the probability of a hypothesis, the Bayesian probabilistic specifies some prior probability, and then updates it in the light of new data. The Bayesian interpretation provides a standard set of procedures and formulas to perform this calculation.

[36]PNNL. *Validation of Statistical Sampling Algorithms in Visual Sample Plan (VSP): Summary Report*, PNNL-18253 (Richland, Wash.: February 2009).

and achieved the desired confidence levels (to within acceptable tolerances). DHS provided us estimates of funding for external validation of the VSP software algorithm by an independent third party, however, such funding is not currently available, according to DHS.

According to the developer, although the combined judgmental and random sampling approach was developed for site characterization and clearance purposes, it could also be used for initial sampling. NIOSH evaluated the combined judgmental and random sampling approach in an internal full-scale exercise in December 2010. According to HHS, while NIOSH did identify many challenges in using it during this exercise, the primary outcome of the discussion of the NIOSH field exercise was a determination of whether this sampling approach would be useful for future investigations. It was decided that it was not applicable for general investigations, but would be useful in special cases when levels of confidence in sampling results were needed. Its usefulness in situations other than bio-hazard sampling was also acknowledged.

In HHS's comments on this report, it noted that this approach still requires a fair amount of subjective judgment in selecting input parameters to use the tool and that collecting additional samples will increase costs. According to PNNL, after the exercise, CDC supported PNNL in making additional modifications to the combined judgmental and random modules to better support ease of use and furniture placement. PNNL stated that when judgmental samples do not identify contamination while evidence is strong that contaminations exists, such as in sick people, or that the risk is high, the VSP biological and chemical contamination sampling modules would prove beneficial and most likely necessary even though locating randomly selected sample locations would prove more difficult than it would for judgment samples. (Appendix IV describes how the combined judgmental and random sampling approach could be used.)

Composite Sampling

In March 2012, EPA officials stated that statistical confidence statements are difficult to make with judgmental sampling results. However, EPA often collects composite samples—that is, uses the same collection device at more than one location—allowing it to collect from the same number of locations with fewer sample numbers. If statistical sampling requires 100 samples from 100 locations, composite sampling can cover the same number of locations with 25 samples (1 sample covering 4 locations), reducing the number of samples by a fourth as well as the time. One problem, however, with composite sampling, according to CDC and EPA, is that if a sample is positive, then all surfaces sampled in that composite sample should be considered positive. Also, if any composite sites are contaminated, contamination can be spread to uncontaminated sites.

However, this problem could be somewhat controlled by collecting composites in an appropriate manner. For example, according to EPA, composite sampling can be conducted room by room. If the whole composite sample (or room) were to test positive, then the entire room would be decontaminated.[37] It is, however, important to note that (1) composite samples do not allow statistical confidence statements, and (2) if decision makers require statistical confidence statements, then a composite sampling approach could not be used.

Building Experiments

DHS conducted two experiments in a vacant building in an Idaho National Laboratory (INL) facility to evaluate, among other things, the combined judgmental and random sampling design.[38] These experiments were intended to demonstrate that a particular sampling approach worked and would generate data helpful to decision makers and also to provide baseline data that would contribute to validation. Neither experiment provided opportunities to evaluate the advantages of statistically-based sampling approaches, including the merits of the combined judgmental and random sampling over judgmental sampling at different levels of contamination, as planned.

The first experiment failed to meet its objectives regarding the sampling approaches because of cross-contamination by the simulant that was released. The second experiment failed to meet some of its objectives, including its objective to evaluate and compare probabilistic and the combined judgmental and random sampling approaches for clearance in a building with gradient contamination—including low and no

---

[37]That is, if any composite sample—taken in whole or in part—from a room were to test positive, then the entire room would be subject to decontamination.

[38]Validation of the overall process involves designing experiments that demonstrate that the sampling approach works to develop executable sampling plans to meet decision makers' needs, according to DHS. The draft strategic plan states that developing and executing a sampling plan experiment will enable validation of the overall process of constructing and executing sampling plans under the guidance of the sampling strategy document.

contamination.[39] According to an independent evaluation of the second building experiment, even though the contamination density decreased from the first to the second building experiment, the sampling approaches could not be differentiated by their detection rate or overall recovery.[40] However, the detection rate in the second experiment was about 40 percent and more. Testing at only high contamination density, however, does not address situations of low levels of contamination.[41]

VSPWG agencies differed in their opinions on certain aspects of these experiments and their ability to adequately evaluate the sampling approaches. According to an EPA official, a gradient of contamination was achieved in the second building experiment, and it was found that "judgmental sampling results were 'as good as' those generated by statistical sampling."[42] According to HHS, while judgmental sampling cannot provide specified levels of confidence in findings, except possibly when based on confidence in the investigator's expertise, "confidence" is subjective.[43] Further, HHS stated that with regard to the building experiments, differentiating between the probabilistic and judgmental sampling approaches depends on sample sizes and a determination of confidence levels in results.

Sampling approaches are needed that have a greater chance of identifying low levels of B. anthracis. A future release of B. anthracis spores, according to the independent evaluation of the second experiment, could take place in many different scenarios. For example, it

---

[39]The second building experiment had several objectives. For sampling approaches, they were to (1) operationally evaluate judgmental and probabilistic sampling for characterization and (2) evaluate and compare probabilistic and the combined judgmental and random sampling approaches for clearance in a building with gradient contamination (from low or moderate down to absent or not detectable) for different initial concentrations of the contaminant.

[40]See Jeffrey H. Grotte and Margaret Hebner, *Operational Observations on the INL-2 Experiment,* IDA Paper P-4449 (Alexandria, Va.: August 2009).

[41]We did not independently verify these data.

[42]According to EPA, these experiments showed that judgment sampling identified all contaminated locations but with a much smaller number of samples compared to statistical sampling. This appears to relate to the objective: operationally evaluate judgmental and probabilistic sampling for characterization.

[43]NIOSH apparently conducted focus groups that according to HHS supported this assertion. We have not seen the results of these focus groups.

might involve a (1) low concentration of agent, (2) a small amount of agent might be efficiently aerosolized, (3) a small portion of a larger amount might be aerosolized by inefficiencies of dispersion, or (4) a larger amount might be aerosolized in a space larger than the building used for the second experiment.

Probabilistic sampling approaches must be based on appropriate models of contamination, and the data (or numbers of trials) must be relevant for determining the pattern and quantity of sample that should be collected to identify contamination, according to an expert we consulted. However, the study conditions in the second experiment were such that the observed contamination patterns did not match the desired gradient and localized contamination patterns.

To evaluate the VSP biological contamination sampling module performance against the judgment-sample-only option, the contaminated area would ideally have been a small area, since the VSP module is set up to ensure a high probability that at least one contaminated sample will be obtained if some small percentage of the surface area is contaminated, according to PNNL. Combined judgmental and random sampling was used for the clearing sampling plan, including clearing during the characterization phase of an area that was planned to be uncontaminated. However, because contamination was found (positive result), confidence statements regarding the absence of detectable contamination could not be made. Therefore, issues regarding judgmental and probabilistic sampling approaches remain unresolved.

Before an experiment, pretest studies can be used to evaluate such things as dissemination efficiency or settling characteristics before deciding the amount of simulant to be disseminated. For example, according to an expert we consulted, information from pretest studies on dissemination amounts could have been used to revise the experimental design for the second building experiment before it was implemented so that the amount of simulant released would have been more likely to result in a gradient of contamination—areas of both high and low contamination. Areas of low contamination are needed in testing probability-based sampling approaches. DHS has stated that pretest studies had been conducted for the building experiments to guide an understanding of what might happen in the test.[44] However, according to PNNL, these studies were not adequate, with the bigger issue being the failure to reduce the amount of contaminant released.

DHS has also stated that the building experiments were expensive and that it was technically difficult to release a known but very low concentration that would adequately test combined judgmental and random sampling. We recognize that VSPWG has learned from the problems experienced during the two building experiments with respect to sampling approaches. Nevertheless, in future experiments, as stated by the expert we consulted, concentration gradients may not be achieved until appropriate studies have been conducted with simulant in the facility in which the simulant is to be released for testing purposes.

VSPWG's Validation Studies on Methods Are Not Yet Complete

CDC, EPA, and the FBI would each have a unique role in a bioterrorism incident, but their methods have many commonalities for initial sampling, environmental characterization, and evidence sampling, even though they have different goals. These agencies would benefit greatly if they used validated methods, regardless of who validates them.

The environmental sampling methods the FBI used to respond to the 2001 *B. anthracis* attack were not validated. Since the FBI's mission is not environmental monitoring, however, VSPWG member agencies that perform environmental sampling take the lead in developing and validating methods for environmental sample collection. DHS has now established the NBFAC, whose accredited laboratory supports law enforcement forensic requirements. The FBI primarily relies on NBFAC to validate its microbial forensic analytical methods. NBFAC currently has

---

[44]These studies involved the dissemination of polystyrene beads before the actual simulant tests to determine the amount of material to be released and to identify the conditions needed to achieve the desired dissemination results during the tests. Also, in a 2011 building experiment, according to HHS, pretest studies ensured that a gradient concentration was established.

several ISO 17025 accredited analysis methods for identifying and characterizing *B. anthracis*.[45]

CDC and EPA have stated that the FBI has its own analytical methods and does not typically use CDC's and that while the devices may be similar, the methods are not exactly the same. Determining whether differences between the FBI's analytical methods developed by NBFAC and those of CDC and EPA are significant might be useful. NBFAC is not involved in validating collection methods. Therefore, improvements in sample collection procedures or protocols, including those for the swab, wipe, and vacuum, could be useful to the FBI in developing its sampling plans, regardless of how heavily contaminated an area is. (See appendix V for more information on the FBI's methods.)

According to experts we consulted, validating a method involves selecting and using a collection method and device, transporting the collected samples to a laboratory, preparing them for analysis, and then analyzing them at that laboratory. Each step must be validated in a laboratory where confounding variables can be controlled. A complete validation study addresses all procedures in the process where variation could occur. For example, variation could occur because of surface collection methods, conditions of transportation, or preparation and analysis.

Validation studies typically provide information on the following performance parameters: accuracy, limit of detection, limit of quantitation, linearity, intermediate precision (variability within laboratories), precision (variability between laboratories), range, ruggedness, sensitivity, specificity, false positive and false negative rates (inferred from percentage specificity). A validating entity may quantify all parameters applicable to the methods being validated. Ideally, validation would include quantifying the performance measures for each step to understand the total uncertainty. However, this could be difficult to

---

[45]The FBI will obtain useful information on the strengths and weaknesses of LRN-validated methods through its membership in VSPWG. It will also be able to compare them and make improvements where necessary to its own environmental sampling methods. CDC and EPA have stated that the FBI has its own methods and does not typically use those that CDC developed and that while the devices may be similar, they are not exactly the same. However, an FBI official told us that the FBI has done side-by-side comparisons of collection methods, including LRN's, which if they prove superior, will be adapted for the FBI. It noted that it has access to methods other than those LRN developed.

achieve, and jointly quantifying all the sources of variation could be sufficient. Alternatively, quantifying some sources of variation together and some separately, depending on the methodology, might be sufficient. (These parameters are defined in appendix VIII.)

Three Completed Studies	CDC has validated two preparation and analysis methods—the swab and wipe. In addition, PNNL and SNL have conducted a study of CDC's wipe method.

CDC's Swab Study

CDC has validated the macrofoam swab for the preparation and analytical methods in a laboratory environment but not for sample collection or transport.[46] It has stated that all steps in collection, transport, preparation, and analysis cannot be separated for validating environmental samples. According to CDC, evaluating these steps independently is not possible since the only way to determine how effective the first two steps are (collection and transport) is to use the second two steps (preparation and analysis). CDC stated that it would be difficult to attempt to validate the swab collection method in the field and that traditional industrial hygiene method development does not require it. CDC further stated that reducing and defining individual variations in collection methods is better approached through training, in post-training, and in evaluation during competency assessments under simulated field condition in a laboratory setting.

Even though validating the swab collection method in the laboratory might be challenging, it can be done. We agree with CDC that collection cannot be validated in a field study because controlling for several confounding variables would be difficult. We also believe that validating storage and transport issues is not as critical when dealing with *B. anthracis* spores— they are hardy organisms able to withstand varied conditions without loss of viability—compared to more delicate organisms, such as viruses.

---

[46]CDC conducted laboratory studies on the swab method in 2007 and the wipe method in 2009 and published studies on the LRN validation. It also posted the swab procedures on its website in 2008 and the wipe procedures in 2010.

For the swab, the 2010 laboratory study focused on the variability of the preparation and analysis methods:

1. To collect samples, CDC personnel used pre-moistened macrofoam swabs to wipe surfaces (steel coupons) that had previously been inoculated with *B. anthracis* Sterne spores;

2. CDC personnel then packaged and shipped (overnight on cold packs) the collected swab samples to the 12 LRN laboratories that participated in the study, where samples were processed within 48 hours;

3. Personnel at these laboratories prepared the samples for analysis by extracting spores from them (by vortexing), and then analyzed them using culture and PCR.[47]

CDC's validation study for the swab evaluated various performance parameters under various levels of spore contamination for the preparation and analysis methods. The study evaluated accuracy, limit of detection, limit of quantitation, linearity, precision (reproducibility-variation between laboratories), intermediate precision (variability within laboratories), range, sensitivity, specificity, and false negative rate (inferred from percentage specificity).[48]

CDC noted that ruggedness was demonstrated by the use of different analysts, instruments, and reagent lots throughout the study. Thus, the CDC study for the macrofoam swab presents results for preparation and analysis on these parameters. According to CD documentation, the study did not address robustness (variation in method parameters) and one aspect of precision (that is, repeatability: same conditions over a short interval of time).[49]

---

[47] Appendix VI has more information on the swab study.

[48] See L. R. Hodges, L. J. Rose, H. O'Connell, and M. J. Arduino, "National Validation Study of a Swab Protocol for the Recovery of *Bacillus anthracis* Spores from Surfaces," *Journal of Microbiological Methods* 81 (2010):141-46, and L. R. Hodges, L. J. Rose, A. Peterson, J. Noble-Wang, and M. J. Arduino, "Evaluation of a Macrofoam Swab Protocol for the Recovery of *Bacillus anthracis* Spores from a Steel Surface," *Applied and Environmental Microbiology* 72 (2006): 4429-30.

[49] In the study, only one shipment per inoculum level was evaluated.

The study also did not quantify the false negative rate as a function of other variables. In commenting subsequently on the draft report, HHS stated that robustness was inherent in the validation study and that deliberately introducing variables in the study was not necessary since variables were built into it. That is, each participating laboratory used different models of instruments to conduct the processing, according to HHS. Further, CDC did not conduct extensive evaluations for recovering low numbers of spores to acquire the false negative rate, noting that this work was not funded and SNL was to conduct a study.[50] DHS planned to fund PNNL and SNL to conduct a study of the CDC swab method to generate data on false negative rates and other performance parameters. However, according to DHS, this study has been delayed for lack of funding. (See also appendix VI for information on studies on the methods.)

CDC's Wipe Study

Similarly, for the cellulose sponge wipe method, CDC has validated the preparation and analysis methods in a multi-laboratory study, but not collection or transport. CDC stated that all steps could not be separated for validating environmental samples. CDC reiterated the difficulties it believed it would encounter in attempting to validate wipe collection in the field and in the laboratory, as it would for the swab method. CDC also does not intend to conduct a validation study of the wipe collection method in a laboratory setting. However, as stated previously, CDC prefers to address variations in collection methods through training, in post-training, and evaluation during competency assessments under simulated field conditions in a laboratory setting. We believe that validating the wipe collection method in the laboratory would be challenging but possible.

---

[50]False negative rate is a function of other variables, such as the concentration of contaminant, the surface material being sampled, and the specific set of sampling and analysis methods. See also appendix VIII for definitions of the performance parameters.

For the wipe, CDC's 2011 laboratory validation study focused on the variability of the preparation and analysis methods:

1. Two CDC personnel collected sponge-stick samples from previously inoculated steel surfaces that were then shipped to the laboratories participating in the study.[51]

2. At these laboratories, personnel prepared the samples for analysis by extracting spores from the sponge stick samples.

3. Laboratory personnel then analyzed them using culture and PCR.

Regarding collection, the wipe study stated that because it was intended to focus on the variability of the processing method in multiple laboratories, only two individuals collected samples before they were transported to the various laboratories for preparation and analysis. According to the study, this was done to keep variability to a minimum.[52] The study recognized that in an actual sampling event, additional variability could be introduced by multiple individuals conducting the sampling.

The CDC study for the cellulose wipe method presented results for preparation and analysis for the following parameters: accuracy (percentage recovery), limit of detection, limits of quantitation, linearity, precision (reproducibility), intermediate precision (variability between laboratories), range, sensitivity, specificity, and false positive rate (inferred from the percentage specificity).[53] The study did not evaluate

---

[51]Sample collection procedures in the study consisted of CDC personnel using the sterile sponge to wipe across the surfaces in a vertical motion, turning the sponge over, wiping in a horizontal motion, and then using the sides of the sponge to swipe in a diagonal motion across the coupons. The tip of the sponge (held perpendicular to the surface) was then used to wipe around the edges of the coupon to pick up spores that may have been pushed to the edges.

[52]In the swab and wipe studies, CDC personnel collected the samples before transporting them to the participating laboratories, whose personnel then prepared and analyzed the samples they received—as opposed to the participating laboratories' personnel collecting the samples directly from the steel surfaces (coupons). Consequently, the effect of such variation was not factored into the study.

[53]L. Rose and others, "National Validation Study of a Cellulose Sponge Wipe-Processing Method for Use after Sampling *Bacillus anthracis* Spores from Surfaces," *Applied and Environmental Microbiology* 77 (2011): 8355-59.

precision (repeatability, or the same conditions over a short interval of time) or robustness or quantify the false negative rate as a function concentration and surface materials.[54] As it did for the swab, HHS subsequently commented that robustness was inherent in the study since each participating laboratory used a different model of instruments to conduct the processing. They did not conduct extensive evaluations recovering low numbers of spores to acquire the false negative rate, noting that this work was not funded.

PNNL and SNL Wipe Study

At DHS's request, NIST and PNNL reviewed several laboratory studies on the performance of sampling methods using the swab, wipe and vacuums—including the CDC validation studies on the macrofoam swab and cellulose sponge wipe—and identified three major gaps.[55] Generally, these studies did not (1) provide certain information on the performance of sampling methods (for example, the false negative rate); (2) capture all the sources of uncertainty affecting performance results and associated with fully understanding the limitation of the method; and (3) capture all the sources of uncertainty affecting performance results and associated with fully understanding the limitation of the method.[56] All but one of the studies failed to investigate the false negative rate and quantify how it

---

[54]The study noted that the data do not address the potential for variability between multiple shipments, or runs, at the same inoculum level, since each laboratory processed only a single run for each inoculum level.

[55]Many previous studies investigated only short-term, within-test uncertainties (repeatability) and did not investigate run-to-run or laboratory-to-laboratory uncertainties (reproducibility). Thus, they did not include all the relevant sources of variation. Therefore, according to PNNL, the estimates of performance measure uncertainty reported in those studies can be expected to underestimate the total uncertainty. See G.F. Piepel and others, DOE: *Laboratory Studies on Surface Sampling of Bacillus anthracis Contamination: Summary, Gaps, and Recommendations*, PNNL-20910 (Richland, Wash.: November 2011).

[56]NIST stated in May 2012 that the report provides guidance as to recommendations for additional experimental work to support a better understanding of the method performance parameters and characterization of uncertainly. Several of the recommended activities have been pursued by the agencies since 2010, according to NIST, and documentation of their outcomes is cited elsewhere in this report. NIST also stated that since the since the 2010 report, NIST has worked to maintain and expand a literature review of bacterial collection method performance parameters and to develop an understanding of potential contributions to uncertainty. However, NIST stated that the 2010 report was ambitious in its statements on the third gap—that is, the need to capture "all of the sources" of uncertainty. NIST stated it has since worked to gain a better understanding of the critical sources of uncertainty when referring to sample collection method performance.

varies with contaminant concentration level, surface material, and other factors that varied in the studies.

Consequently, DHS funded PNNL and SNL to conduct a study of the CDC wipe method to generate data on false negative rates as a function of surface material and surface concentration of the contaminant, other performance parameters, and their uncertainties.[57]

The PNNL and SNL study on the CDC sponge-wipe method concluded that wide testing of the method was lacking.[58] It noted that the food industry has used sponge wipe methods for decades, and the CDC-validated method is expected to have extensive use in environmental sampling. Further, according to the study, the wipe method had been tested in only one CDC study that did not test the method at lower contaminant concentration levels that may yield false negatives.[59]

The PNNL and SNL study attempted to evaluate false negative response rates as a function of the level of concentration for each of six different surface materials. It evaluated the wipe method by testing with very low concentrations of spores deposited on a variety of nonporous surfaces, followed by surface sampling, preparation, and analysis, using a modified LRN protocol.[60] Specifically, it evaluated the effects of contaminant concentrations and surface materials on recovery efficiency, false negative rates, limits of detection, and the uncertainties of these quantities.

According to EPA, one major issue with this study is that it used liquid inoculation (as in CDC studies) rather than dry dissemination, as was used in the bioterrorism event. This was done so that very low spore

---

[57]See G. F. Piepel and others, DOE: *Laboratory Studies on Surface Sampling of Bacillus anthracis Contamination: Summary, Gaps, and Recommendations*, PNNL-20910 (Richland, Wash.: November 2011), and G. F. Piepel and others, DOE: *Summary of Previous Chamber or Controlled Anthrax Studies and Recommendations for Possible Additional Studies*, PNNL-SA-69338, rev. 1 (Richland, Wash.: December 2010).

[58]See P. A. Krauter and others, "False Negative Rate and Other Performance Measures of a Sponge-Wipe Surface Sampling Method for Low Contaminant Concentrations," *Applied and Environmental Microbiology* 78(3) (December 2011): 846-54.

[59]The SNL study tested spore concentrations of 3.10×10^{-3} to 1.86 CFU/cm^2.

[60]It used the spore simulant *B. atrophaeus,* while the CDC study used the vaccine strain *B. anthracis Sterne.*

concentrations could be applied to a surface and then sampled. According to EPA, the problem with this approach is that very low concentrations of dry material do not behave the same way and can be spread. EPA further stated that the process of collecting a sample could affect the surface concentration. EPA concluded that the study on false negative rates is likely to have underestimated the false negative rates from a dry dissemination.

Regarding sample collection, the PNNL and SNL study generally used the CDC study's procedures for collecting wipe samples on hard, nonporous surfaces in both indoor and outdoor environments.[61] In the study, three technicians were assigned to three steps of the sampling and analysis process (collecting, processing samples, and enumerating results) in a balanced way. According to the study, these balanced assignments protected against confounding any effects of test locations and technicians with the primary test variables (that is, contaminant concentration and surface material).

The PNNL and SNL study on the wipe found that smoother surfaces yielded higher recovery efficiencies and lower false negative rates for the wipe. It concluded that it might be possible to improve sampling results by considering surface roughness in selecting sampling locations and interpreting spore recovery data. It also concluded that gains in performance improvement suggested that the sponge-wipe method was approaching what is required to reliably detect B. anthracis at lower surface concentrations.

In addition, regarding sampling variation, PNNL and SNL also reported that imperfect, less than 100 percent, sampling recovery is common and that the variation in sampling methodology, techniques, spore size and characteristics, surface materials, and environmental conditions will cause variation in recovery efficiencies, false negative rates, and limits of detection. Also, they reported that, according to other studies, the overall recovery efficiency is sensitive to the applied experimental conditions for

---

[61]The study's sample collection procedures were as follows: Using a sterile technique and a sterile, premoistened sponge wipe (or sampling device), each test coupon (or contaminated surface to be sampled) was wiped in an overlapping "S" pattern with horizontal strokes. The wipe was then rotated, and the coupon was wiped with vertical S strokes. The sample area was then wiped in diagonal "S" strokes. Sample collection was concluded by wiping the edge of the surface.

GAO-12-488 Anthrax Detection

a wide range of potential variables in surface sample collection methods, such as differences in extraction solution, adsorptive material, surface substrate, and surrogate biomaterial. Further, spore recovery from a surface is complex for various reasons, including spore characteristics, the environment, the presence of grime or competing microorganisms, sample media, and method. They noted that a way to control these variables was to use standardized methods.[62]

Two Types of Studies Are Needed before Validation Is Complete

Validation will not be complete until VSPWG conducts two types of studies: collection methods in a laboratory setting for the swab and wipe and false negative rates for the swab. Laboratory studies on the collection methods would determine the variation inherent in the physical sampling of a surface with a swab or wipe. Further, studies that address gaps in performance data, including data on uncertainty and false negative rates, have not been completed for the swab.[63] Values for false negative rates must be addressed so that assay measurements depicting reliable low-level or zero residual contamination can be evaluated.

CDC's validation of the swab and wipe in its laboratory studies did not include the collection method, as previously discussed, or quantify the false negative rate as a function of concentration and surface materials. CDC officials stated on March 8, 2012, that methods are never 100 percent validated. The swab and wipe are fit for their purpose—that is, a public health response. CDC stated that it decided that validation of the collection parameter was not realistically feasible, given the infinite variables possible in an actual event. Nevertheless, an important reason why different collection methods have been developed and studied is that some of them are more efficient and reproducible than others. In June 2012, HHS stated that CDC had already fully validated swab and wipe processing and analysis methods for detecting *B. anthracis* in a laboratory setting, which is consistent with the definition of validation

---

[62]Paula A. Krauter and others, *False Negative Rate and Other Performance Measures of a Sponge-Wipe Surface Sampling Method for Low Contaminant Concentrations. Applied and Environmental Microbiology* 78(3) (December 2011): 846-54. See also Da Silva and others, 'Parameters affecting spore recovery from wipes used in biological surface sampling. *Applied and Environmental Microbiology* 77 (2011) 2374-80.

[63]As stated earlier, validating storage and transport issues is not as critical when dealing with *B. anthracis* spores—they are hardy organisms able to withstand varied conditions without loss of viability—compared to more delicate organisms, such as viruses.

under ISO 17025. Nevertheless, as we stated previously, ideally, a laboratory study would address all procedures in the sampling process where variation could occur, including variation from not only the preparation and analysis methods but also the surface collection methods and the conditions of transportation.

A complete validation study would incorporate the collection methods. According to experts we consulted, while it may not be practical to validate collection methods for every operational condition in the laboratory, it is important to determine the influence that collection methods have on the results of a study. Standard sampling protocols have been developed that can be tested to determine how they influence method performance measures discussed previously. However, the designs of the CDC validation studies for the swab and wipe methods did not include a determination of the variation inherent in the physical sampling of a surface. The lack of evaluation of collection in the studies means that its effect on performance parameters such as recovery efficiencies, false negative rates, and limit of detection has not been measured. Consequently, VSPWG's efforts to validate remain incomplete.

While the preparation and analysis methods are important variables, ideally, the swab study would have been significantly more comprehensive if CDC personnel had inoculated the steel surfaces with the spores and then directly transported them to the 12 laboratories participating in the study. This way, different personnel at these laboratories could have collected samples from the steel coupons, prepared the samples by extracting the spores from them, and finally analyzed the spores for a complete validation of the process. However, we recognize that the integrity of the inoculated surfaces could be compromised during transport of the steel surfaces to the participating laboratories. Therefore, an alternative could be CDC's conducting a controlled in-house study with an appropriate number of CDC personnel collecting the samples.

According to VSPWG members, a study similar to that conducted for the wipe to address gaps in performance data, such as the false negative rate as a function of other variables, is also planned for the swab method although funding is not available. In summary, until these gaps in performance characteristics are addressed, validation of the methods will not be complete.

VSPWG's Several Challenges in Completing Validation

Although progress has been made in validating the methods, VSPWG must address several challenges before the validation project can be completed: (1) clarifying the scope of the validation project, updating the strategic plan, and determining VSPWG's future; (2) reaching VSPWG member consensus on the range of sampling approaches that should be available to decision makers; (3) establishing a realistic estimate of time for completing prioritized validation activities; (4) addressing scientific gaps, such as assessing risks without dose-response data; and (5) ensuring that funds are available for completing critical tasks.

The Validation Project's Scope Should Be Clarified

A significant weakness in VSPWG's effort is that it has not updated the 2007 strategic plan to reflect the project's current scope and direction. A validation project of this type requires prolonged and sustained effort. We testified in 2006 that a strategic plan and roadmap can help monitor progress and measure agency performance toward validating *B. anthracis* sampling methods.[64] The roadmap must, however, reflect accurately, to the extent possible, the validation activities that implement the strategic plan, must reliably estimate the time and resources needed to complete them, and must account for any limitations or uncertainties that may affect progress.

However, VSPWG has not yet achieved consensus on what is required to link together all the steps that the 2007 strategic plan indicated were necessary to complete validation, along with others added since the plan was implemented. The need to incorporate sampling results in a risk-based framework is one example. Also, VSPWG will need to determine what further refinements of the sampling approaches and sampling methods are necessary when considering the state of the science regarding the risks that *B. anthracis* contamination poses to those exposed and the intended use of these methods in a future incident. As a result, the strategic plan might not reflect the direction in which the project is currently headed.

Revisions and adjustments are expected in long-term projects like this one, but they should also be reflected in periodic revisions to the strategic plan and its roadmap. Our discussions with agency officials and our

---

[64]GAO, *Anthrax: Federal Agencies Have Taken Some Steps to Validate Sampling Methods and to Develop a Next-Generation Anthrax Vaccine*, GAO-06-756T (Washington, D.C.: May 9, 2006).

review of the documentation provided to us lead us to conclude that the roadmap does not yet reflect all the activities needed to complete validation or indicate what can be validated consistent with ISO 17025. Also, the estimated funding may need further consideration.

A DHS official told us that DHS had intended to revise the 2007 interagency strategic plan. However, in September 2011, DHS stated that discussions with VSPWG members regarding how to complete the project indicated that CDC and EPA preferred to terminate VSPWG. Various reasons were given by VSPWG members. For example, EPA stated, among other things, its concern about the lack of leadership and internal funding. DHS stated that the reasons stemmed from CDC's and EPA's decision regarding the use of judgmental sampling regardless of the circumstances of the incident (discussed in more detail later in this report). Finally, some VSPWG members indicated in March 2012 that they thought that the strategic plan was overly ambitious with goals that were unlikely to be met. A DHS official disagreed, stating in May 2012 that the VSPWG had not maintained the 2010 consensus it had reached in 2007. This official stated that fulfilling the requirements of the strategic plan is hampered by the lack of funding and commitment as well as the shift of attention to wide-area versus indoor contamination.

The strategic plan states that during its execution, revisions are expected, as conditions warrant, to enhance, clarify, and account for unforeseen challenges. Current conditions suggest that the strategic plan and its roadmap, as appropriate, would benefit from revisions, including further clarification of the scope, VSPWG consensus on what is required to complete the project, and a commitment from VSPWG to complete the associated tasks. Also, in view of funding challenges, revised estimates of funds and realistic timelines are needed to ensure completion of the critical tasks that VSPWG decides are necessary to the project. Until these conditions are met, the project's future will be uncertain.

VSPWG Consensus Is Needed to Resolve Outstanding Issues

Consensus among VSPWG members on some remaining disagreements is needed for VSPWG to move forward. Consensus of VSPWG members on the range of sampling approaches that would be available to decision makers during the full range of sampling phases has not yet been reached. The strategic plan addressed sampling and analysis activities related to public health investigation and response to and remediation of known or potential contamination by *B. anthracis* spores disseminated as a powder or aerosol within a facility.

CDC and EPA collect and analyze environmental samples for different purposes—initial sampling and sampling for environmental characterization and decontamination—but use common methods. They are considering how to respond to a wide-area release of *B. anthracis*—a worst-case scenario—outside the scope of VSPWG's validation effort. The 2001 release, described as small-scale, affected primarily indoor environments.[65] CDC has stated that statistical sampling will rarely be used in the future while EPA does not believe it is necessary. Therefore, it is not clear whether an approved statistically-based sampling approach—using combined judgmental and random sampling or another appropriate method—will be available for decision makers to use at their discretion in an incident in which a facility might have low levels of contamination.[66]

CDC advised us that it would use judgmental sampling only in its initial sampling. CDC states that it has successfully used judgmental sampling in several post–2001 *B. anthracis* events reporting anthrax in exposed persons. These were naturally occurring releases of *B. anthracis* unrelated to bioterrorism. CDC officials subsequently stated that CDC would—in limited scenarios involving an indoor release—consider combining judgmental and statistical sampling. According to NIOSH, the combined approach might be used when judgmental samples are all negative and could include, but would not be limited to, the following:

1. other interested parties (unified or incident command, political leaders, public health agencies, building owners) requesting a specified level of confidence that the area of concern is free of contamination or

2. intelligence or strong medical evidence (such as confirmed cases of anthrax linked to a location) points to a high risk of contamination in the location.

---

[65]Alexander G. Garza, MD., MPH, Assistant Secretary for Health Affairs and Chief Medical Officer, Department of Homeland Security, written statement before the Senate Committee on Homeland Security and Governmental Affairs, "Ten Years after 9/11 and the Anthrax Attacks: Protecting against Biological Threats?" Washington, D.C., October 18, 2011.

[66]As we have stated, combined judgmental and random sampling is intended for characterization or clearance sampling but could be used for initial sampling purposes if a decision maker decided that statistical confidence statements about contamination were needed in a particular situation.

For the rare circumstances in which CDC uses statistical sampling during the initial response, limitations would include the availability of qualified staff, personal protective equipment, and sampling supplies while maintaining situational awareness as the event unfolds. CDC would also need to maintain capacity to rapidly conduct judgmental sampling at other sites. HHS has stated that statistically-based sampling would be labor and resource intensive and could affect response times, processing more samples than are needed to adequately assess risk.

EPA has shifted its planning and preparedness approach for biological incidents, placing a priority on a wide-area urban *B. anthracis* incident. EPA officials told us that this is a worst-case scenario similar to national planning scenario 2—a release of aerosolized *B. anthracis,* with both outdoor and indoor contamination.[67] EPA's sampling approach for characterization and decontamination, according to EPA officials, will be site- and incident-specific and will favor judgmental sampling. EPA intends to apply its approach to both wide-area release scenarios and those like the indoor release in 2001. EPA officials told us in March 2012 that given EPA's current budget and what it believes is operationally practical in responding to a wide-area release, it will make site- and incident-specific decisions but is likely to rely on judgmental sampling in federal buildings, followed by wide-scale decontamination.[68] EPA officials told us that the agency has always used judgmental sampling for reasons of operational reality, laboratory capacity, and cost. EPA has characterized its approach as risk management, acknowledging that it cannot eliminate all risk but would rather strive to reduce as much risk as possible, according to EPA officials.[69] EPA's and CDC's clearance goal is

---

[67]National Response Framework, Department of Homeland Security, Scenario 2: Biological Attack—Aerosol Anthrax (Washington, D.C.: January 2008).

[68]EPA has also cited presidential directives and DHS planning scenarios in its decision to refocus planning on worst-case scenarios. Regarding nonfederal buildings, EPA has said that it will offer technical guidance to building owners and local public health officials who have ultimate responsibility for determining whether a building should be decontaminated and whether it is safe for occupancy.

[69]According to EPA officials, EPA relies on multiple lines of evidence in making cleanup and decontamination verification decisions, including epidemiological information, data from judgment sampling, data from decontamination technology parameter measurements (decontaminant concentration, contact time, temperature, humidity), data from biological indicators such as spore strips (as was done with the Senate Hart office building in 2001), data from decontamination technology efficacy studies, and modeling of the areas of potential contamination.

currently no detectable, viable spores, following post-decontamination sampling.[70]

CDC and EPA have acknowledged that after a response to a wide-area release, viable residual spores may be present below the current sampling and analytical detection limits, in both indoor and outdoor environments. However, the infectious dose is currently unknown, which is important when considering people who may have compromised immune systems (such as the elderly) that make them vulnerable to disease. Thus, reliance on medical countermeasures is expected in order to ensure that exposed persons do not become ill. Stating that it is ultimately up to property owners and the lead public health agency whether buildings will be decontaminated in a wide-area release, an EPA official told us that the agency will decide how to approach each case from site-specific information. However, according to EPA, in a wide-area release, local public health agencies and an Environmental Clearance Committee (an independent group that would include representatives from EPA and other agencies) would give advice.[71]

Disagreement about the merits of a validation activity in the 2011 roadmap addressing statistical issues has also arisen. CDC and EPA officials have told us that as the use of probability sampling is now rare, they object to two related activities in the 2011 roadmap.[72] However, a DHS official told us that completing this activity has merit. Further, according to DHS, completing the overall validation effort fulfils the

---

[70]See CDC and EPA, *Interim Clearance Strategy for Environments Contaminated with Bacillus anthracis* (Washington, D.C.: February 2012).

[71]This committee, to be formed in the event of a release, would be an independent group of experts. Groups that might be represented on the committee could be the local, county, or state public health agencies; facility or property owners; and local government and subject matter experts from CDC, EPA, and OSHA. The committee would conduct a comprehensive review to evaluate the effectiveness of decontamination efforts. Ultimately, it would base its recommendations on whether clearance goals had been met and decontaminated areas could be reoccupied.

[72]These two activities are listed in the 2011 roadmap as "statistical sampling and confidence formulas." Tasks include extending formulas to account for the false negative rates with two statistical sampling approaches. The total cost for the statistical sampling activity and the confidence formula activity is estimated to be $951,000.00 and $540,000.00, respectively, according to the February 2011 funding data provided to us. According to PNNL, tasked with completing this work, a report summarizing the first phase of the "confidence formula" work is nearly done. The remaining work is to further improve the combined judgmental and random sampling approach.

commitment made in the 2006 memorandum of understanding. Statements regarding assessment of "cleanliness" or absence of contamination should be scientifically defensible, and scientifically valid explorations of the technical issues of sampling and analysis—which VSPWG has been conducting—should include such studies. According to DHS, whether predominantly statistical sampling is rare is irrelevant to the need to describe uncertainty associated with it. EPA officials stated in March 2012 that the federal budget is not unlimited for investing in research for an approach unlikely to be employed when other critical gaps in *B. anthracis* response go unfunded, such as data on dose response effects that possibly could allow a more liberal clearance goal.[73] However, DHS stated in May 2012 that it would be funding these two activities.[74]

DHS, as chair of VSPWG, has indicated that it believes it is compelled to complete its commitment as expressed in the 2006 memorandum of understanding and explore the GAO's 2005–06 suggestions. The current scope of validation project is for a small-scale, indoor release. In May 2012, EPA stated that whatever approach VSPWG develops for an indoor release should apply also to a wide-area release when more than one building is contaminated and health risk concerns are the same as or less than some others.

A DHS official stated In September 2011 that DHS would like to complete VSPWG's current roadmap task regarding indoor sampling with combined judgmental and statistical sampling, stating also that wide-area sampling is not within VSPWG's scope and noting that the indoor and wide-area contamination scenarios should not be confused. Several VSPWG members indicate that if they reach no agreement, the project will end. Regardless of the decision, CDC and EPA officials have indicated to us that both agencies will complete their designated tasks in the roadmap if funding is available. Nevertheless, it is still not clear how continued disagreement on probability-based sampling as a discretionary tool for

---

[73]Such gaps, according to EPA, include data on spore fate and transportation, re-aerosolization, and dose response effects that possibly allow a more liberal clearance goal; greater knowledge of decontamination efficacy, capacity, and capability; greater laboratory capacity and capability; and enhanced data management tools. EPA would use them in responding on a regular basis; filling these gaps is relevant for both low- and high-contamination incidents.

[74]Delays in completing these activities stem from funding decreases rather than overall expenses or technical challenges, according to DHS.

decision makers will affect the outcome of this project or VSPWG makeup.

Agencies and decision makers in a small-scale attack would benefit from having the option of using an approved probability sampling approach. *B. anthracis* still heads the list of threat agents. However, we recognize that in an external environment—as in a wide-area attack—more confounding factors weigh, as a practical matter, against using statistically-based sampling. Nevertheless, although a decision to use probabilistic sampling in a given situation might be rare, as CDC has acknowledged, some situations may warrant a specified level of confidence.

Further, EPA has expressed interest in having a more user-friendly version of the VSP software available whereas CDC believes such investment is not necessary. EPA stated in May 2012 that PNNL has not created a user-friendly version that would enable federal responders to use the VSP software with ease—presumably in either type of response. CDC stated in May 2012 that it already had a software model that it could use in such rare situations when considered appropriate. CDC noted that while this product could benefit from further refinement, it is functional for limited public health needs. Further development is not necessary.

In contrast to CDC, EPA has suggested that, under a commitment to DHS, PNNL deliver a user-friendly version of the software, sent as a final deliverable product to CDC, DHS, and EPA. Should other evidence during an investigation raise questions about the potential for contamination in areas that were not originally sampled, the availability of an approved statistical sampling approach for decision makers to use at their discretion—that is also operationally feasible for those using it—seems reasonable to us.

Validating the Methods on Time May Be Challenging	Completing all validation activities in the 2011 roadmap was scheduled for the end of fiscal year 2013, but this milestone is not likely to be met because of challenges facing VSPWG. Some key tasks remain, and further delays may occur because of other agency priorities—as happened with the CDC and EPA responses to the H1N1 outbreak and the Deepwater Horizon incident. Also, according to DHS, prioritization of activities generally occurs as a group consensus, and funding is not necessarily strongly correlated with priority.

Studies on the performance gaps, such as the false negative rates versus concentration curves, are planned for the swab and vacuum (should a candidate be found and validated by CDC) and transport methods.[75] CDC stated in June 2012 that it is focusing its efforts on evaluating several different vacuum sampling methods to identify a suitable method for future laboratory validation work involving porous surfaces. Data on most of the relevant performance parameters for the swab and wipe preparation and analysis methods have been collected. Laboratory studies on the collection methods would ensure a complete validation of the swab and wipe methods. VSPWG will have to focus on completing these critical tasks first. In a future incident, these methods will provide results that decision makers rely on. CDC, according to the 2011 roadmap, still has to conduct multi-center validation of transport and storage procedures, although as previously stated, these procedures are less critical for *B. anthracis*.[76] However, we recognize that comprehensive validation of all methodologies is not possible.

Addressing Scientific Gaps Will Be Difficult in the Short Term

Sampling approaches (such as judgmental and statistical), the sampling methods, and validation of those methods, need to be seen in the context of what they are to achieve. Public health initial sampling is primarily done to detect the event and characterize the agent, and epidemiologists assess the risk of exposure, help define who may have been exposed, determine potential pathways of exposure to support the epidemiological investigation, and also support decisions related to medical treatment, according to CDC. Risk assessment should include hazard identification, exposure assessment, dose-response assessment, and risk characterization, according to the National Academy of Sciences (NAS). Thus, data from sampling would likely be one of the factors used to develop risk assessments.

---

[75]According to PNNL, although PNNL and SNL have been asked to provide estimates for testing and experimental design and data analysis for the swab, this work has not yet been funded or started because of DHS's science and technology budget cuts.

[76]In addition, CDC has to evaluate vacuum methods for sampling porous surfaces, and EPA has to validate the Rapid-viability PCR method. CDC officials told us on March 8, 2012, that they had begun to evaluate several vacuum methods to determine whether any could be candidates for further study and eventual validation. Therefore, it is unclear when this evaluation will be completed or indeed whether a suitable candidate will be found. EPA officials told us in March 2012 that its validation of the Rapid-Viability PCR method will depend upon further research in fiscal years 2012-13 and the availability of required funding. EPA anticipates conducting multilaboratory validation of this method with selected sample types and eventual publication.

However, CDC has told us that data do not exist that link levels of surface contamination with a quantitative risk for inhalation anthrax in humans. Identifying the extent of contamination, although necessary for identifying potentially exposed individuals and for decontamination, cannot be used to determine the risk for humans of developing anthrax disease through inhalation since the infectious dose for susceptible individuals is not known.

The risk relates not just to the level of contamination but also to the extent to which spores may—under particular circumstances—be transferred from contaminated surfaces to cause inhalation or cutaneous anthrax. This is still not well understood despite some limited studies. According to a 2009 study that included CDC, DOD, and EPA collaboration, developing a standard for a presumably safe level of surface contamination requires an understanding of the rate at which spores on surfaces become aerosolized.[77] According to this study, some limited research has been conducted into inhalation infectivity but estimates of the lethal dose vary. Further, limitations of relating exposure to inhalation infectivity include quantification of the ability of spores to move from a surface and become re-aerosolized, quantification of exposures of the resulting aerosol, uptake by exposed humans, and room size and ventilation characteristics and exposure time, according to the study.

In 2001, of the 22 people who became ill with clinical anthrax, half had inhalation anthrax (5 of whom died), while the others had cutaneous anthrax. The investigation concluded that some of those who had inhalation anthrax had been exposed to re-aerosolized spores from contamination on surfaces. Nevertheless, the study concluded that despite these limitations concerning health risk, standardizing the performance of surface sampling methods is necessary.

Another study also addressed the lack of understanding of inhalation anthrax resulting from animal and human exposures.[78] It stated that in 2001 policy makers and risk managers did not have access to scientific

[77]C. F. Estill and others, "Recovery Efficiency and Limit of Detection of Aerosolized *Bacillus anthracis* Sterne from Environmental Surface Samples," *Applied and Environmental Microbiology* (2009): 4297–306.

[78]M. E. Coleman and others, "Inhalation Anthrax: Dose Response and Risk Analysis," *Biosecurity Strategy, Practice, and Science* (2008): 147–59.

evidence—dose-response data. Understanding dose-response relationships and the underlying mechanisms of disease resistance are essential for effective risk management and preparedness planning, according to this study.

Absence of data on the infectious dose in exposed individuals leaves no basis for determining whether a certain contamination level in fact poses a health risk and, thus, whether certain remedial actions (for example, decontamination) are appropriate, according to our experts. Consequently, further refinements of sampling methods and their validation raise questions about whether their results will provide information useful for supporting decision makers—unless policy dictates that any level of contamination is a concern.[79] If so, the better the quality of information about the level of contamination generated by sampling, the more likely that there will be an appropriate response—even for low levels of contamination.[80]

While we may have a well validated method, it is essential to also know the relationship between the level of contamination indicated by use of that method and what that means for those who have been exposed to it. Because this information is still lacking, the relevant question remains: Is this facility contaminated? As a result, the reliability of the sampling methods is significant in a response. Therefore, the real question is, Has a sufficient job of validating these methods been done so that one can be confident about their capabilities?

Ensuring That Funds Are Available for Completing Critical Tasks

DHS acknowledged in July 2011 that it was difficult to say whether funds would be available to complete the activities, noting that the validation project has lower agency priority. Also, according to DHS, funding by participant agencies is generally within each agency's program prioritization schemes. Further, prioritization of activities generally occurs as a group consensus, and funding is not necessarily strongly correlated with priority.

---

[79]For clearance purposes, the goal is no viable detectable spores.

[80]In defining low-level contamination, agencies are likely to base levels on their experience; "low" is likely to include the number and distribution of samples needed for confidence in a negative (that is, nondetected) finding as well as the elusive health-risk element associated with levels of contamination.

Validation of the methods for sample collection, transport, preparation, and analysis will be completed as funds, personnel resources, and competing priorities permit, according to DHS. This will be challenging for the scarcity of funding in VSPWG agencies' program budgets from budget cuts. While the 2011 roadmap projected completion of the validation activities by the end of fiscal year 2013, DHS now anticipates that this milestone will not be met because of recent cuts to VSPWG agency budgets and competing agency priorities. Total funding obligated or planned for VSPWG activities for fiscal years 2005–13 was estimated at $16.3 million in February 2011. Funding for fiscal years 2005–11 was about $11.6 million of this amount. Estimated funding for fiscal years 2012–13 is about $4.7 million and subject to availability. Of the project's total $16.3 million, each activity's total ranges from $100,000 for sample integrity studies to about $5.6 million for collection and analysis method studies. The collection and analysis methods (34 percent), field experiments (22 percent), and performance gap studies (16 percent) constitute the largest percentages of funding. Smaller percentages include validation of the combined judgmental and random module at about 7 percent and confidence determination and statistical methods development at about 9 percent. External independent review and overall process validation is projected to be about 9 percent. (See appendix VII for more information on the project funding.)

Conclusions

Federal agencies were not prepared to respond to *B. anthracis* contamination on the scale of the *B. anthracis* attack in 2001. While several agencies, with unique expertise and missions, responded to the incident, no one entity could coordinate the multiagency response. Because the agencies lacked scientifically validated detection methods, not much was known about the performance characteristics of the methods they used at that time and how they might have affected the results (positive or negative). When the results were negative, the judgmental sampling agencies used in their initial sampling did not allow them to make a confidence statement regarding whether a building was contaminated.

Using only judgmental sampling is a concern, particularly in a scenario where contamination could be low and test results are negative. Therefore, we concluded in 2005 that the negative results of the testing of the postal facilities in 2001 presented uncertainties because of the limitations associated with the agencies' sampling methods and approaches. While neither judgmental nor probabilistic sampling is guaranteed to produce positive results in the presence of low-level contamination, a statistically-based sampling approach will allow decision makers to make statistical confidence statement regarding the likelihood that a building is contaminated. Appropriate validated statistical models will give additional capabilities to decision makers. Internal validation of the VSP model for combined judgmental and random sampling has already been completed, and DHS plans to fund external validation of this model. Thus, when fully validated, a reliable statistically-based sampling approach will be available to decision makers, should a situation warrant its use.

Under the interagency strategic plan and roadmap, the DHS-led VSPWG agencies have taken several actions to respond to our recommendations. Their activities were intended to validate the environmental sampling methods and to develop a statistically-based sampling approach that allows confidence statements, an important achievement. From the progress since 2001 in validating sampling methods for detecting *B. anthracis* spores in indoor environments, more is now known about the performance characteristics of the swab and wipe methods from CDC's validation studies on the preparation (extraction) and analysis methods and the PNNL and SNL study to quantify false negative rates for the wipe method.

Moreover, the FBI relies on NBFAC to validate its analytical methods for microbial forensics, which is outside VSPWG's scope, but it also looks to the lead agencies that validate environmental sampling methods. Consequently, it benefits from any improvements in sample collection procedures or protocols for the swab, wipe, and vacuum because they are useful to the FBI when it develops its sampling plans or evaluates its environmental sampling methods.

However, CDC does not intend to validate the collection methods for the swab and wipe in either controlled laboratory studies or field studies. While we agree that controlling for confounding variables in field studies would be difficult, we disagree with CDC on its position regarding laboratory studies, where one can control the confounding variables. CDC has stated that its collection procedures have demonstrated through training exercises and real world exercises that they are fit for its purpose. However, the point of validation is to determine where variation in the process is significant so that special emphasis can be directed to training in those areas.

Nevertheless, because of the variables in collection, we believe that not validating these methods for the swab and wipe leaves the assessment of process (collection, preparation, and analysis) incomplete. Even though validating the collection methods may be challenging, it could be done in a laboratory setting, perhaps in an in-house study to mitigate the effects of transporting samples to other laboratories. The study designs for the swab and wipe did not include a methodology for determining the variation inherent in physically sampling a surface. Less critical is validation of transportation methods because *B. anthracis* spores are hardy. Other aspects remain to be studied: additional studies on the false negative rates have been completed for the wipe but delayed for the swab for lack of funding. Until all these studies have been conducted for the swab and wipe, we believe validation of these methods will not be complete. Because these methods continue to be the mainstay of sampling indoors in myriad environments, validating collection and learning more about the false negative rates with different contaminant levels are worthwhile.

Although progress has been, and continues to be, made regarding validation of *B. anthracis* detection methods, VSPWG faces several challenges. The scope of the project needs clarification. Some VSPWG members think that the strategic plan is overly ambitious and its goals unlikely to be met and, therefore, wish to terminate the work group. In contrast, DHS thinks a greater obstacle is members' impatience with the lack of progress because of decreased funding for tasks as well as the shift of attention to the wide-area contamination issue. DHS believes also that sampling is implicitly tied to a risk-based decision process made on the basis of sampling results, while others disagree.

We understand that DHS may wish to pursue these important issues but the strategic plan needs to be revised so that it is more explicit in this regard. Further, VSPWG has agreed to present in its guidance a range of sampling approaches that decision makers could use in an incident, without favoring one over another. Nevertheless, it has not yet reached consensus on whether additional work should be done to improve statistically-based sampling modules so that they could be more operationally feasible in a future incident. While DHS is willing to conduct further work, HHS believes it is unnecessary since statistically-based sampling will be used rarely, and EPA believes a user friendly version should be made available to CDC, DHS, and EPA. Therefore, VSPWG agencies will have to come to a consensus on tasks needed to complete the project and on whether they wish to continue to function as part of the workgroup to complete the agreements made in the 2006 memorandum of understanding.

Nevertheless, the sampling process entails scientific gaps that have not been addressed. Appropriate actions to deal with actual or possible *B. anthracis* contamination of a facility will depend on two factors: the level of contamination and the health risk that any particular level poses. Information on the level of contamination relies for the most part on the results of sampling. Studies on sampling methods will provide information on their performance characteristics. Given the many environmental variables in buildings and other indoor environments, and especially in the field, however, comprehensive validation of all methodologies is not possible. Nevertheless, it is essential that when data about contamination are provided to decision makers, some evaluation of the statistical reliability of such data should be included. This is particularly important in the case of low-level contamination when test results may be negative even though contamination is present.

The human health risks from any particular level of exposure still remain uncertain too. The effectiveness of both sampling approaches and sampling methods must be considered in the context of what they are required to achieve, such as support for decisions about the risks that contamination poses and subsequent actions. Further refinement of sampling methods and sampling approaches without such clear goals risks unproductive research and development.

DHS indicated in May 2012 that it continues to pursue completion of the validation project. However, we recognize that obtaining funding for the remaining activities in the project will mean that VSPWG agencies will have to compete for such funding with other agency priorities within broader agency programs. Consequently, the time for completing the project will need to be readjusted to establish more realistic milestones should the VSPWG agencies reach consensus on unresolved issues and agree to continue to move forward as an interagency workgroup sharing its resources. It must be emphasized that CDC's and EPA's data and advice on sampling will be relied on by decision makers who have to make difficult decisions in emergency situations. Thus, their sampling data need to be the best. Also, they will need to understand and communicate the limitations of those data.

Finally, we recognize that the VSPWG has attempted to address a difficult task involving validating sampling methods for *B. anthracis* and exploring alternative sampling approaches. Since the workgroup has invested about $12 million and considerable resources over about 7 years, it would be prudent for it to work toward agreement and complete prioritized tasks. Thus, the workgroup may wish to consider carefully what work is needed and think strategically in terms of its investments and their potential benefits.

Recommendations

To ensure that federal agencies have validated sampling methods for detecting B. anthracis in indoor environments and—in the case of negative results—the option of using appropriate sampling approaches to make statistical confidence statements about the likelihood that a building is free of contamination when potentially there has been a low-level release, we recommend that the Secretary of Homeland Security take steps to complete the validation project. Statistically-based sampling designs for such purposes would encompass any sampling with a statistical basis, including a probabilistic only approach as well as one that combines judgmental and probabilistic sampling. Achieving a sufficiently rigorous validation of the sampling methods and ensuring that statistically rigorous and mutually acceptable sampling approaches are available will provide options that will better prepare decision makers to respond to a future bioterrorism incident.

DHS should

- update the strategic plan and its roadmap with an agreed-on scope and revised timelines and

- complete the validation project, including validating the collection methods in a laboratory setting in a manner that determines the potential sources of variation in collection method performance, including variation that could be introduced by individual samplers, and related ongoing studies.

We also recommend that the Secretary of the Department of Health and Human Services and the Administrator of the Environmental Protection Agency support DHS in its goal of achieving (1) validated sampling methods to understand the limitations of the data that would be provided to decision makers, and (2) a mutually acceptable statistically-based sampling approach that can be employed when decision makers—such as Incident Commanders and others—conclude that statistical confidence statements need to be made about the level of contamination in a particular indoor environment.

At the end of our review, after we had submitted the draft report to the agencies, issues were raised regarding the specific intent of our recommendations that in turn led to further communication with DHS,

HHS, and EPA. As a result, we revised our recommendation to clarify our intent. The recommendations stated in the draft report sent to the agencies were as follows: DHS should (1) update the strategic plan and roadmap with an agreed-on scope and revised timelines; and (2) complete the validation project, including validating the collection methods and completing ongoing studies. Also, HHS and EPA should support DHS in its goal of achieving validated sampling methods and a mutually acceptable statistically-based sampling approach that can be employed in those situations in which decision makers—such as Incident Commanders and others—conclude that statistical confidence statements need to be made about the level of contamination in a particular environment. Eventually, we revised the recommendations to those stated at the beginning of this section.

Agency Comments and Our Evaluation

We obtained written comments on a draft of this report from DHS, EPA, and HHS. Their comments regarding our recommendations are printed in appendixes IX–XI. We discuss their key concerns below. In addition, DHS, DOE (PNNL), EPA, the FBI, HHS, and NIST provided technical comments that we have addressed in the body of our report where appropriate.

DHS agreed with our recommendations, and EPA and HHS generally disagreed with them. DHS agreed with our recommendation that it update the strategic plan and roadmap with an agreed-on scope and revised timelines. DHS stated that the DHS-led VSPWG had developed a consensus roadmap in August 2011 that will be revised to reflect appropriate scope as well as to recognize subsequently delayed milestones caused by funding losses in agency programs. Additionally, DHS stated that it intends to update the strategic plan to reflect advances the group has made since 2007 and the remaining tasks toward achieving the goals participating agencies jointly agreed to in the 2006 interagency memorandum of understanding. However, DHS noted that the support of EPA and HHS will be essential to completing this update.

DHS also agreed with our recommendation that it complete the validation of the collection methods—in a laboratory setting in a manner that determines potential sources of variation in collection method performance, including variation that could be introduced by individual samplers—and also completing ongoing studies. DHS stated that it intends to fulfill its obligations as described in the 2006 memorandum of understanding. Further, DHS stated that it believes that incident commanders should have well-founded options for conducting sampling campaigns in contaminated structures and appreciates GAO's recognition of its efforts to outline and characterize those options. Both EPA and HHS agreed to support DHS in updating the strategic plan and roadmap. EPA agreed to complete validation efforts as appropriate. HHS also agreed that additional work is needed to address gaps in B. anthracis sampling strategies and methods.

However, HHS did not agree with our recommendation that it support DHS in achieving validated sampling methods to understand the limitations of the sampling data provided to decision makers and completing ongoing studies. HHS stated that there is no need to validate collection methods under controlled conditions in a laboratory to determine potential sources of variation attributable to multiple samplers. Rather, HHS believes that reducing and defining individual variation in collection methods is better approached through training, in post-training evaluations, and during competency assessments under simulated field conditions in a laboratory setting.

We believe that validating collection methods under controlled laboratory conditions will establish information—based on a best-case scenario—on a selected set of variables. It will also provide data that, while not applicable to an actual event, would more fully characterize the method and thus expectations of how it will perform in an actual event. We recognize that the CDC laboratory validation studies of the processing (preparation) and analysis methods for the swab and wipe have provided needed information on their performance parameters, as has the additional PNNL and SNL study on the wipe. However, in the absence of validation of collection, it is not clear to what extent the accuracy of the results will be affected when contamination is close to the threshold level of detection.

Further, while training and competency assessments of collection methods are important practices, they will not take the place of laboratory validation. The point of laboratory validation is to determine what variation exists in the process—including collection—so that data generated by that process can be provided to decision makers along with communication of its limitations. Laboratory validation will also identify areas of significant variation so that special emphasis can be directed to training in those areas to improve technician performance. HHS contends that training and competency assessments in the laboratory would address this issue, but this statement could also be made for the extraction and analysis procedures, which would in effect negate the need for the study.

Human technicians are responsible for sampling spores from surfaces. The techniques applied during the sampling process (for example, overlapping "S" patterns with horizontal strokes, and rotating the coupon and wiping with vertical "S" strokes) will certainly vary from technician to technician, and these variations must be characterized to quantify the accuracy of the entire process. Accordingly, training can make operators more consistent in their collection technique, but it cannot change the physical and chemical properties of the collection device itself. Therefore, technician training, while valuable, cannot overcome the naturally inherent variation from the physical and chemical properties of the process.

Both EPA and HHS disagreed with our recommendation that they assist DHS in reaching its goal of achieving a mutually acceptable, statistically-based sampling approach that can be employed in situations in which decision makers—such as incident commanders and others—conclude that statistical confidence statements need to be made about the level of contamination in a particular indoor environment.

EPA stated that a statistically-based sampling approach is not needed from a science perspective and is not possible with today's realities. EPA stated that there are larger gaps that need to be filled to address *B anthracis* decontamination. For an alternative to our recommendation, EPA recommended that it develop a policy paper that clearly explains how confidence statements can be made when using targeted, or judgmental, sampling approaches, combined with additional sampling-related information (for example, weighting based upon incident specific information) and approaches (for example, composite sampling methods or new, validated sampling).

We believe that only sampling approaches with a statistical basis allow confidence statements. Targeted, or judgmental, sampling approaches, by themselves, are not sufficient in situations in which statistical confidence statements are required.

This view is reflected in an EPA guidance document.[81] For example, EPA's guidance states that whether to use a judgmental or statistical

---

[81]See EPA, *Guidance on Choosing a Sampling Design for Environmental Data Collection for Use in Developing a Quality Assurance Project Plan*, EPA QA/G-5S (Washington, D.C.: December 2002). www.epa.gov/quality/qa_docs.html.

(probability based) sampling approach, is a main sampling design decision.

Also, EPA's guidance states that

> "An important distinction between the two types of designs is that statistical sampling designs are usually needed when the level of confidence needs to be quantified, and judgmental sampling designs are often needed to meet schedule and budgetary constraints."

Limitations of judgmental sampling, according to this guidance, are that "Judgmental sampling does not allow the level of confidence (uncertainty) of the investigation to be accurately quantified."

Importantly, statistical sampling approaches are not limited to purely random samples that do not allow for scientific knowledge or professional judgment. A well designed statistical sampling approach incorporates expert scientific judgment as well as site-specific circumstances. This approach is also reinforced by EPA's guidance, which states that the

> "Implementation of a judgmental sampling design should not be confused with the application of professional judgment (or the use of professional knowledge of the study site or process). Professional judgment should always be used to develop an efficient sampling design, whether that design is judgmental or probability-based."

Moreover, without statistically-based sampling, the test results will be qualitative and, more importantly, there could be instances when contamination might be missed and the consequences are unpredictable. In a crisis, it would be hard to tell a decision maker that agencies believe an area is free of contamination but that the certainty of that belief cannot be determined. That is, agencies cannot quantify the confidence levels for the results provided to them. Alternatively, agencies must make it clear that when they use judgmental sampling, their negative results have limitations, including an inability to provide a quantitative estimate of the likelihood of contamination. In the future, there will undoubtedly be unique situations in which judgmental sampling alone will not be sufficient for a decision maker's needs.

Both EPA and HHS expressed concerns about the resources and costs associated with statistical sampling. Specifically, EPA stated, the environmental laboratory analytical capacity that would be needed does not exist for a statistically-based sampling approach and neither does the manpower to support sampling, or the software to handle the data without significant, costly investments. HHS stated that statistical sampling is labor and resource intensive, exhausting capacity and detracting from the overall government response at times when rapid response is most critical. HHS is concerned that applying this approach would dramatically affect response times and inappropriately direct much-needed resources to collecting and processing more samples than are required to adequately assess risk.

We agree that statistical sampling would generate a larger sample size; thus, it would be resource intensive and costly compared to judgmental sampling. However, we are not recommending indiscriminate use of this approach. Rather, we are recommending that a validated, statistically-based sampling approach be available for discretionary use by decision makers in situations in which the risk of not using such an approach outweighs any concerns about its cost. We recognize that implementing a statistical sampling approach would affect laboratory capacity. A laboratory may not be able to analyze all the samples on a given day.

However, several potential solutions include (1) not analyzing all samples, once collected, on the same day (given that *B. anthracis* spores do not deteriorate while in acceptable storage conditions in a laboratory) and (2) increasing laboratory capacity by hiring more staff for the existing laboratories and transporting the samples for analysis to more than one laboratory. In situations where the level of contamination is low, if agencies were to decide to use only judgmental sampling and test results were negative, they must recognize that they could lose a number of days if they decide to collect additional samples. Consequently, critical time for public health interventions would be lost.

Regarding the number of samples required to adequately assess risk, as we reported, VSPWG members differ on whether exploring the relationship between sampling results and risk management is within the scope of the project. However, assessing risk is one of the realities of sampling that decision makers must face in an incident. Thus, for decision makers, the lack of a validated, statistically-based sampling approach for use in the rare circumstances when additional steps are needed undermines agencies' overall preparedness.

In heavily contaminated areas, we agree that judgmental sampling would be efficient and economical. We are only suggesting that statistically-based sampling be used when decision makers decide a statistically-based confidence statement is necessary. Such circumstances could include those in which vulnerable populations (young, elderly, sick) have potentially been exposed. This could apply in indoor and wide-area (indoor-outdoor) contamination, and we agree with EPA that the decision to use this approach in one building over another could be politically sensitive. Nevertheless, the option needs to be available. Further, while we accept that there are gaps in decontamination, our focus is on initial sampling.

EPA also stated that it is concerned that we continue not to recognize that the overall response on Capitol Hill was successful using targeted (or judgmental) sampling and that studies such as INL's continue to reenforce the effectiveness of targeted sampling. We agree that judgmental sampling usefully allows for expert scientific judgment and for site-specific circumstances to be considered in determining the location and the number of areas to sample. We also agree that judgmental sampling approaches have proven successful in identifying contamination when applied to incidents in which areas are heavily contaminated, such as on Capitol Hill and in the Brentwood Postal Facility. In this regard, we have recognized in our report that in cases in which contamination levels are high, there is no need for statistical sampling. However, in the two studies conducted at INL, conditions were not adequate to evaluate judgmental and statistical sampling approaches in buildings with low levels of contamination—a circumstance in which decision makers could decide to use statistically-based sampling.

With respect to sampling approaches that should be available to decision makers, we agree with DHS that they should have well-founded sampling options, and we believe that a statistically-based sampling approach is a necessary tool when statistical confidence statements are required—even if they rarely are. In this report, statistically-based sampling encompasses any sampling with a statistical basis, including a probabilistic-only approach and one that is a combined judgmental and probabilistic approach. We also recognize that appropriate sampling plans must consider the response phase (initial assessment, characterization, clearance) and should use judgmental, statistical, and combination sampling approaches. As we stated, our concern is focused on initial assessment in a building where contamination could be low, decisions are being made whether to conduct additional sampling in light of the circumstances (such as a potential for exposure of immune-compromised individuals), knowledge about a release at a particular site is not definitive, or illness has been reported despite negative results from initial sampling. It is important to remember that decision makers in a future incident will rely on CDC's and EPA's expertise and capabilities when making difficult decisions. The agencies' detailed responses follow.

HHS stated that scientifically defensible sampling approaches are needed (for example, targeted, or judgmental, and statistical sampling approaches) that can inform incident commanders and other decision makers with critical information, including limitations of the procedures and estimates of confidence limits. In support of its conclusion, HHS stated the following:

HHS stated that CDC has successfully used targeted, or judgmental, sampling approaches to identify contamination in several post 2001 *B. anthracis* events. For example, it used a targeted approach in the 2009 New Hampshire investigation that successfully identified levels close to the levels of detection of contamination in the building of concern. As we have stated, judgmental sampling approaches are both effective and economical, particularly when definitive information is available. These *B. anthracis* events were natural occurrences—not covert or intentional releases—in which information was available and some of those exposed to the spores were diagnosed with anthrax disease. Since positives were found using a judgmental approach, and contamination was identified during initial sampling, there was no need to do statistical sampling. Only when initial sampling does not reveal low-level contamination and certain conditions are present—such as increased diagnoses of illness that suggest that spores are present—would the judgmental sampling approach need to be reconsidered. Further, we do not believe that HHS can extrapolate from CDC's success in these limited scenarios that its methodology has been developed to the point where it can handle any future event, including scenarios we have not considered or do not believe are possible.

HHS noted that circumstances are rare in which HHS and CDC would consider using statistical sampling during the initial response but that using statistical sampling is limited by the availability of qualified staff, personal protective equipment, and sampling supplies for conducting the sampling. It is limited too by the need to maintain situational awareness as events unfold and to maintain the capacity to rapidly conduct targeted sampling at other priority sites as they are identified. HHS also stated that CDC has a software module for statistically-based sampling in the rare circumstances when it is required. HHS stated that this module could benefit from further refinement, but it is functional for the limited public health needs and further development of statistical approaches is not necessary.

We recognize that deciding to use statistical sampling would have to take into account the limitations that HHS has outlined. We also understand that using a statistical sampling approach will most likely be rare.

However, EPA has suggested that a user-friendly version of the sampling module be made available to DHS, EPA, and HHS. Finally, DHS states that such a tool should be available to decision makers, and it intends to externally validate the combined judgmental and random statistical model, although funds are not currently available. It is clear that if a method that is to be used while it is functional, it should also be operationally feasible. Thus, further discussions between the parties could determine the way forward on this issue.

Finally, we believe that despite the challenges it has faced, the VSPWG has made great progress in characterizing the methods and exploring various sampling approaches. We recognize that current budget cuts and competing priorities will require difficult choices. Nevertheless, we believe that in updating the strategic plan and coming to consensus on some differing opinions will serve to move the project to its conclusion and will help improve preparedness capabilities of agencies whose actions or advice will be critical to decision makers in a response to a future incident.

As agreed with your offices, unless you publicly announce the contents of this report earlier, we plan no further distribution until 30 days from the report date. At that time, we will send copies of this report to interested congressional committees; the Secretary of Homeland Security, Secretary of Health and Human Services, and Administrator of the Environmental Protection Agency; and others who are interested. The report is also available at no charge on the GAO website at www.gao.gov.

If you or your staff have any questions about this report, please contact Timothy M. Persons, Ph.D. at (202) 512-6412 or personst@gao.gov. Contact points for our Office of Congressional Relations and Office of Public Affairs appear on the last page of this report. Key contributors to the report are listed in appendix XII.

T.M. Persons

Timothy M. Persons, Ph.D.
Chief Scientist

Appendix I: Objectives, Scope, and Methodology

Our objectives were to identify (1) the extent to which the Department of Homeland Security (DHS) has addressed our recommendations, (2) the extent to which the environmental sampling methods for detecting *B. anthracis* spores in initial public health sampling and microbial forensic investigations have been validated, and (3) any challenges remain to completing validation.

To determine the extent to which DHS's actions have addressed our recommendations, we assessed the evidence on their validation activities DHS and Validated Sampling Plan Working Group (VSPWG) agencies provided. We identified VSPWG actions that have responded to the issues we identified in our 2005 report, as well as DHS's coordination and monitoring of VSPWG's activities. To do this, we reviewed and analyzed, among other things, VSPWG documentation, including the 2006 interagency memorandum of understanding, signed by CDC, DHS, EPA, and NIST; 2007 interagency-agreed strategic plan and its periodically updated roadmaps; ISO 17025; sampling guidance document; and other guidance documents; VSPWG meeting minutes; external review panel assessments and independent assessments of building experiments; validation studies; and funding data for and management of the validation project, among others.

To determine the extent to which the environmental sampling methods applied in public health and microbial forensic investigations have been validated, we compared the definition of validation VSPWG adopted to guide its activities to the agencies' processes for validating methods.

To determine the extent to which the environmental sampling methods applied in public health and microbial forensic investigations for detecting for *B. anthracis* spores during initial sampling have been validated, we reviewed the definition of validation the DHS-led VSPWG)—adopted to guide its validation of the sampling methods. We assessed the extent to which the VSPWG agencies have completed the individual activities in the strategic plan's roadmap, including the sampling methods. We did not independently verify the data the agencies collected. Further, we interviewed officials regarding the validation of the environmental sampling methods from with the U.S. Department of Health and Human Services (HHS), the Centers for Disease Control and Prevention (CDC) and its National Institute for Occupational Safety and Health (NIOSH) and the National Center for Emerging and Zoonotic Infectious Diseases; the Environmental Protection Agency (EPA), U.S. Department of Homeland Security (DHS), and National Institute of Standards and Technology (NIST). We visited the Pacific Northwest National Laboratory (PNNL) to obtain further information on some of its validation activities in the roadmap as well as on the Visual Sampling Plan (VSP) software and its chemical and biological sampling modules, including the combined judgmental and random sampling approach.

Regarding the extent to which FBI's environmental sampling methods for microbial forensic investigations have been validated, we reviewed and analyzed documentation the FBI, DHS, and the National Bioforensic Analysis Center (NBFAC) provided to us, as well as other pertinent documentation we identified during our review, including empirical studies and reports on the methods and approaches the federal agencies, including the FBI, used for sampling facilities in the 2001 *B. anthracis* attack. We also interviewed officials of DHS, DOD, the FBI, NBFAC, and NIST regarding validation of the microbial forensic methods, including the environmental sampling methods used in the 2001 investigation. In addition, we visited NBFAC and the FBI Laboratory at Quantico, Virginia, to better understand the development and validation of microbial forensic methods.

We identified challenges to completing the validation that the VSPWG agencies have encountered. We reviewed interagency VSPWG documentation, including VSPWG meeting minutes; external review panel assessments; and independent assessments of building experiments, validation studies, and funding data. We also interviewed officials from within HHS: CDC, NIOSH and the National Center for Emerging and Zoonotic Infectious Diseases; DHS, DOD, EPA, the FBI, and NIST to identify challenges to the validation of the methods. Finally, we asked scientists with expertise in public health and microbial forensic investigations to review and comment on a draft of our report. They included James Bristow, M.D., Deputy Director for Scientific Programs, DOE Joint Genome Institute; George V. Ludwig, Ph.D., Deputy Principal Assistant for Research and Technology, U.S. Army Medical Research and Materiel Command; Jack Melling Ph.D. (retired), Former Director, U.K. Centre for Applied Microbiology and Research, Porton Down; Jeff Mohr, Ph.D. (retired), Chief, Life Sciences Division, U.S. Army, Dugway Proving Grounds; and Suresh D. Pillai, Ph.D., Professor of Microbiology and Director, National Center for Electron Beam Research, Texas A&M University.

We conducted our work from March 2010 through June 2012 in
accordance with generally accepted government auditing standards.
Those standards require that we plan and perform the audit to obtain
sufficient, appropriate evidence to provide a reasonable basis for our
findings and conclusions based on our audit objectives. We believe that
the evidence we obtained provides a reasonable basis for our findings
and conclusions based on our audit objectives.

Appendix II: Select Agents and Toxins

The biological agents and toxins listed here have been identified as having the potential to pose a severe threat to both human and animal health, plant health, and animal or animal products. An attenuated strain of a select agent or an inactive form of a select toxin may be excluded from the requirements of the September 19, 2011 Select Agent Regulations.

Agency	Agents and toxins
Department of Health and Human Services	Abrin
	Botulinum neurotoxins
	Botulinum neurotoxin producing species of *Clostridium*
	Cercopithecine herpesvirus 1 (Herpes B virus)
	Clostridium perfringens epsilon toxin
	Coccidioides posadasii/Coccidioides immitis
	Conotoxins
	Coxiella burnetii
	Crimean-Congo haemorrhagic fever virus
	Diacetoxyscirpenol
	Eastern Equine Encephalitis virus
	Ebola virus
	Francisella tularensis
	Lassa fever virus
	Marburg virus
	Monkeypox virus
	Reconstructed replication competent forms of the 1918 pandemic influenza virus containing any portion of the coding regions of all eight gene segments (Reconstructed 1918 influenza virus)
	Ricin
	Rickettsia prowazekii
	Rickettsia rickettsii
	Saxitoxin
	Shiga-like ribosome inactivating proteins
	Shigatoxin
	South American Haemorrhagic Fever viruses

Agency	Agents and toxins
	Flexal
	Guanarito
	Junin
	Machupo
	Sabia
	Staphylococcal enterotoxins
	T-2 toxin
	Tetrodotoxin
	Tick-borne encephalitis complex (flavi) viruses
	Central European Tick-borne encephalitis
	Far Eastern Tick-borne encephalitis
	Kyasanur Forest disease
	Omsk Hemorrhagic Fever
	Russian Spring and Summer encephalitis
	Variola major virus (Smallpox virus)
	Variola minor virus (Alastrim)
	Yersinia pestis
Overlap	*Bacillus anthracis*
	Brucella abortus
	Brucella melitensis
	Brucella suis
	Burkholderia mallei (formerly *Pseudomonas mallei*)
	Burkholderia pseudomallei (formerly *Pseudomonas pseudomallei*)
	Hendra virus
	Nipah virus
	Rift Valley fever virus
	Venezuelan Equine Encephalitis virus
USDA Plant Protection and Quarantine	*Peronosclerospora philippinensis (Peronosclerospora sacchari)*
	Phoma glycinicola (formerly *Pyrenochaeta glycines*)
	Ralstonia solanacearum race 3, biovar 2
	Rathayibacter toxicus
	Sclerophthora rayssiae var zeae
	Synchytrium endobioticum
	Xanthomonas oryzae
	Xylella fastidiosa (citrus variegated chlorosis strain)

Agency	Agents and toxins
USDA Veterinary Services	African horse sickness virus
	African swine fever virus
	Akabane virus
	Avian influenza virus (highly pathogenic)
	Bluetongue virus (exotic)
	Bovine spongiform encephalopathy agent
	Camel pox virus
	Classical swine fever virus
	Ehrlichia ruminantium (Heartwater)
	Foot-and-mouth disease virus
	Goat pox virus
	Japanese encephalitis virus
	Lumpy skin disease virus
	Malignant catarrhal fever virus (Alcelaphine herpesvirus type 1)
	Menangle virus
	Mycoplasma capricolum subspecies *capripneumoniae* (contagious caprine pleuropneumonia)
	Mycoplasma mycoides subspecies *mycoides* small colony (*Mmm* SC) (contagious bovine pleuropneumonia)
	Peste des petits ruminants virus
	Rinderpest virus
	Sheep pox virus
	Swine vesicular disease virus
	Vesicular stomatitis virus (exotic): Indiana subtypes VSV-IN2, VSV-IN3
	Virulent Newcastle disease virusa

Source: NSAR website, www.selectagents.gov.

Appendix III: A Framework for Sampling Design

The objective of sampling is to strike an economic balance between the cost of a census, or the full measurement of all places or objects, and the accuracy of results obtained when a smaller sample of such locations is collected and measured. A difficulty in considering a sampling plan is that the accuracy of results is affected by two types of errors: sampling error (because a sample was not collected and measured for all locations), and nonsampling error (errors impacting the collection and other processing activities). For example, measurement errors such as false negatives from laboratory analysis of the samples are nonsampling errors. To address this complexity in selecting a sampling plan to determine contamination by biological agents in buildings, or the like, we provide a framework to describe the process.

If the subject of investigation (room, building, etc.) can be divided into essentially N distinct small areas that can be clearly identified or located and measured or observed, then the analyst has N elemental sample locations from which to select a subset—that is, the sample locations. The statistical theory and principles used to guide the selection of locations (simple random, cluster, or stratified sampling, cut off census, etc), and the sample size n (number of locations) is referred to as the sampling approach in this report. The collection and the measurement method (how the presence of subject material at each location will be determined) make up the sampling method. The sampling approach and the sampling method make up the sampling plan.[1]

The complexity of the sampling plan becomes apparent. Taking a sample of locations contributes sampling error that must be considered in decision making. Sampling error is the deviation of quantified results for each sample from the quantified results if all locations were in the collection (as with a census of the locations). Further, the measurement at each location may be subject to error—that is, the measurement method does not always produce a value that is precisely true for that location. Measurement error is one type of nonsampling error. Other types of nonsampling error include coverage error, which occurs when

---

[1] In practice, a sampling plan includes such things as the number and type of samples to be collected, the locations from which they are to be collected, how samples will be collected, packaged, and transported to the laboratory, the laboratory or laboratories that will analyze samples; the laboratory procedures and protocols that will be followed in handling, processing, and analyzing samples; the laboratory's quality-assurance procedures; and how it will document and report the results, and management of the data, and health and safety plans.

GAO-12-488 Anthrax Detection

some locations are inaccessible for collection of a sample, and loss or destruction of collected samples.

In deciding on a sampling plan, the analyst must consider both sampling and nonsampling error. A very accurate measurement method might be very costly, making a large sample size unaffordable or too expensive relative to the risk of incorrect decisions based on the results of the sample. But taking too small a sample size in order to contain costs, allow fewer but more accurate measurements, or save time might raise the sampling error to a level such that detecting trace amounts of suspect material has an unacceptable sampling error—that is, low confidence.

For each location in the population, it is possible to collect information by a method (e.g., swab, sponge, vacuum) to be called the sample collection. The material collected needs a transportation method (delivery to the laboratory or intermediate delivery sites), preparation method (the processing of the collected material into a form functional for laboratory analysis) and then an analysis method (quantification of the material to determine the presence or absence of suspect material from the laboratory procedures).

Appendix IV: The Combined Judgmental and Random Sampling Approach

In this appendix, we describe how the combined judgmental and random sampling approach in the Visual Sample Plan (VSP) software, a joint PNNL-NIOSH effort, could be used in a response to an event.[1] Work zones would be set up according to the level of contamination to control access, limit the spread of contamination, delineate areas where personal protective equipment is required, and determine the need for health and safety protocols for entering and leaving those zones, according to the 2010 sampling strategy guidance. For example, a sampling plan could be developed and the potentially contaminated site could be classified as one of four zones:

1. definitively contaminated: evidence is found in a specific location;

2. high likelihood of contamination: initial assessment suggests a plausible

3. pathway;

4. low likelihood of contamination: for example, borders a zone 2 location; and

5. unlikely to be contaminated: for example, is neither contiguous to nor linked with areas bordering zone 2.

A response team should have some a priori belief about the probability of zone 3's being contaminated before assigning it a probability of contamination.

The team should then determine how much more likely it is that the judgmental sample locations are contaminated than other possible

---

[1]As previously noted in this report, the VSP is a software tool that is made up of many sampling design modules, such as those for soil, groundwater, sediments, surfaces, and unexploded ordnance site characterization. VSP's development has been supported by several federal agencies. Specifically, the developer—PNNL—created modules containing sampling approaches that will allow confidence statements by a decision maker, that is, the VSP biological and chemical contamination modules. These modules include probability-based statistical sampling designs and the algorithms pertinent to within-building sampling that allow an investigator to prescribe or evaluate confidence levels of conclusions based on data collected as guided by the statistical sampling designs, according to PNNL. In this report, we refer only to pertinent modules, primarily the combined judgmental and random sampling approach. For more information on VSP, see http://vsp.pnnl.gov/description.stm.

probabilistic sample locations. Figure 5 gives an example of a combined judgmental and random sampling design for a priority area 3 zone.

Figure 5: VSP Screenshot of Combined Judgmental and Random Sampling Module

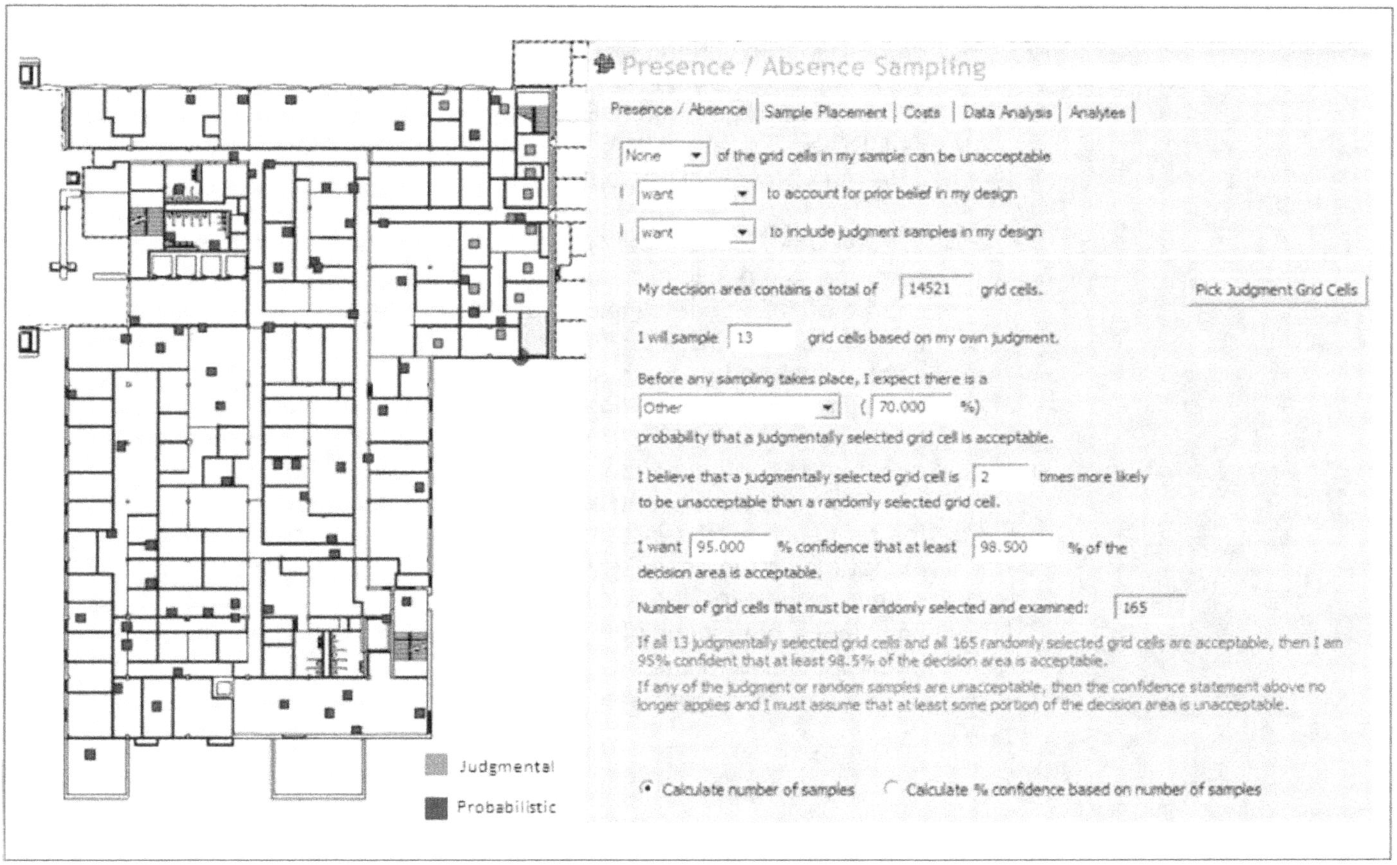

Source: PNNL

Note: This example supports a 95 percent confidence level that at least 98.5 percent of the surface area is below a detectable (or acceptable) contaminant level if all sample results are acceptable. Results are interpreted as either the presence or absence of contamination. The size of the area to be divided into grids is indicated, as is the belief that the area has only a 30 percent probability of containing detectable contamination (70 percent probability that the area is acceptable). In this design, it was decided to collect 13 judgmental samples. The user selected a confidence level, after which the VSP indicated that 165 additional random samples should be collected to obtain this confidence level. Specifically, if none of the 178 sample results are unacceptable (contaminated), there is 95 percent confidence that at least 98.5 percent of the grid cells in the selected area do not contain detectable contamination.

Appendix V: Microbial Forensic Investigations' Objectives Differ from Public Health's

A criminal investigation that involves a microbial forensics investigation may begin in a variety of ways, including such as the discovery of a suspicious powder or a diagnosis of an illness and information from subsequent public health initial sampling. Sampling potentially contaminated buildings also starts with a sampling plan and ends with an analysis of samples at the LRN. However, the FBI may use laboratories other than those in the LRN including the NBFAC, CDC, or other suitable laboratories depending on sampling requirements and availability of resources and personnel. Both the FBI and public health agencies, such as CDC and local public health, and environmental characterization by EPA may be collecting samples simultaneously.

In 2001, the FBI generally used environmental sampling methods common to a public health initial sampling or environmental characterization sampling but for different objectives—to link the material to a source and track down the perpetrator. For example, it collected swab, wipe, and vacuum samples, as did CDC, EPA, and others who participated in the investigation. The FBI told us that it used its sampling methods for two basic purposes: to (1) determine the presence or absence of contamination in areas not known to be contaminated and (2) quantify contamination in areas known to be contaminated. It stated that the presence or absence sampling is analogous to remediation sampling in that maximum sensitivity is desirable, as is confidence in negative results.[1] However, it noted that such sampling is conducted with full knowledge of the limitations of the sampling method and the importance of the sampling location.

---

[1]In contrast to quantifying contamination that has already been found, presence or absence sampling is a qualitative result, indicating only whether spores are present in a sample.

Table 4: The FBI's Sampling Methods

Method	Description	Use
Swab		
Macrofoam, dry	Dry macrofoam swab.	To collect spores in a dry state for preservation and examination from a surface known by prior sampling to be heavily contaminated
Macrofoam, premoistened	ASD Biosystems Sample Collection Recovery Device (SCRD) premoistened with phosphate-buffered saline (PBS) or PBS-Tween. Device has a macrofoam paddle swab attached to lid of 50-ml conical tube; HMRU specified key features to the manufacturer in 2002	Used on smooth or porous but not rough surfaces
Rayon, minitip (male urethral swab)	Supplied dry; wet with PBS before use on dry surfaces	Used in spaces too small for standard swab tip, including gas, water, and electrical fittings in biological safety cabinets
Rayon, standard tip (Q-tip type)	Copan two-tube system with PBS or PBS-Tween 80 wetting agent; made for HMSRU by special order	Used on smooth or porous but not rough surfaces, usually in corners, crevices, and small areas and inside mail bags
Wipe		
Rayon	Supplied dry, aseptically moistened with 1 ml H$_2$O or PBS and inserted into 50 ml conical tube before use	Used on larger smooth surfaces of varying shapes
Vacuum		
Vacuum filter	3M Trace Evidence Filter	Used on broad flat porous surfaces, such as carpet or other rough materials
Other		
Contact plates (RODAC)	Contains special-order formulation of 5% sheep blood agar in TSA with 50 mg/ml polymyxin B sulfate (Becton Dickinson)	Used on flat, smooth, and porous surfaces, including tile, desktops, mail slots, carpet, and cloth; used in known contaminated areas to examine contamination patterns and when rapid culture results are desired
Swab to plate	Moistened Copan Rayon swab	Surface sampled with swab, then used to inoculate standard Petri dish in hot zone; inoculated dish transported to laboratory; used in known contaminated areas when rapid culture results are desired

Source: FBI data.

The FBI also used analytic methods common to those of public health agencies.[2] For example, it conducted traditional microbiological tests on the collected samples to determine (1) whether viable evidence cultures were B. anthracis and (2) using multi-locus tandem repeat analysis, whether outbreak isolates (both clinical and environmental) were the same type of B. anthracis as was used in the 2001 B. anthracis attack— that is, Ames, the strain found in the letters containing the spores.[3] CDC also used this method in its epidemiological investigation.[4] According to CDC, in addition to linking cases, molecular subtyping was useful in determining whether B. anthracis isolated from around the world during the same period was related to the U.S. outbreak in 2001, although these are not LRN approved methods.[5] While it was not validated under the LRN, performance of this method (multilocus tandem repeat analysis) was verified during the investigation by an FBI contractor laboratory and validated afterward by DHS's NBFAC.

The FBI also modified its environmental sampling methods to resolve issues related to the criminal aspects of the investigation, thus, distinguishing its sampling objectives from those of public health's or environmental characterization. For example, it devised a sampling approach to identify other contaminated letters beyond those that had already been found and to track down the mailboxes from which the contaminated letters had been mailed. The FBI used a contact Petri dish to examine patterns of dispersal in the AMI building in Florida. It also used a mini-swab for sampling in spaces too small for the standard swab tip, such as in gas, water, and electrical fittings in biological safety cabinets.

---

[2]The methods are not exactly the same as LRN's, according to CDC.

[3]The genotype was determined with a multiple locus variable number tandem repeat analysis, a method that had been developed for genotypic analysis of B. anthracis before the 2001 attacks. See P. Keim and others, "Multiple-Locus Variable-Number Tandem Repeat Analysis Reveals Genetic Relationships within Bacillus anthracis," Journal of Bacteriology 182 (2000): 2928–36.

[4]A. R. Hoffmaster, C. C. Fitzgerald, E. Ribot, L. W. Mayer, and T. Popovic, "Molecular Subtyping of Bacillus anthracis and the 2001 Bioterrorism-Associated Anthrax Outbreak, United States," Emerging Infectious Diseases 8:10 (Oct. 2002): 1111–16.

[5]HHS notes that molecular subtyping and genome sequencing are not LRN methods for typing the strain of B. anthracis or identifying genetic materials that promote survival.

In contrast, the other agencies were interested in treating those who might have been exposed and, ultimately in remediation—characterizing, decontaminating and clearing the environment of the contamination. FBI investigators also used traditional methods but for different purposes. They used premoistened swabs (in the Trenton facility), HEPA vacuum, and bulk samples in sampling in certain postal facilities and other locations. In its mailbox sampling, for example, the FBI undertook a lengthy process using traditional sampling techniques and laboratory analysis to identify the mailbox from which the contaminated letters had been mailed. Thus, while the FBI worked alongside the public health agencies, benefiting from information gained from their sampling and epidemiological investigation, its sampling was focused on finding evidence that would lead it to a perpetrator of the attack and ultimately to a conviction in a court of law (see table 5).

Table 5: The Objectives of Microbial Forensic Environmental Sampling Compared to Those of Public Health Initial Sampling and Environmental Characterization Sampling

Location	FBI (microbial forensic)	CDC (public health) and EPA (characterization)
AMI building, Fla.[a]		
Objective	To examine contamination patterns to determine how *B. anthracis* had moved through the building and whether a contaminated letter had arrived there	To confirm the source of the first victim's exposure to *B. anthracis* and identify its extent in the building
Analysis	• The FBI, assisted by CDC's Agency for Toxic Substances and Disease Registry, entered the building more than 550 times, removing nearly 5,000 pieces of evidence, including more than 800 letters contaminated by *B. anthracis*.[b] Of 278 samples, many of which were FBI samples collected prior to EPA sampling at AMI, 32 samples were positive for the presence of *B. anthracis* spores • CDC and the FBI returned to the AMI building in summer 2002 to collect additional samples. The FBI had developed a methodology for tracing distribution patterns of *B. anthracis* throughout the 3-story, 68,000 sq. ft. office space. It hoped to use information on the concentration of spores that were detected to determine how the *B. anthracis* had moved through the building and possibly identify the contaminated envelope or package that had led to the anthrax disease in the AMI employees. The FBI used, for example, a contact-petri dish to obtain data	• The diagnosis of inhalation anthrax in an AMI employee had previously been confirmed by the Florida Department of Health but the source of the victim's exposure was initially unknown • CDC sent a team to quantify the building's contamination • EPA then took the lead in collecting samples so it could track the contamination in the building and recommend a decontamination approach (remediation) • *B. anthracis* spores were found in 84 locations in the building. Contaminated samples (78 percent) were collected from the first floor, where the mail room was located. On the first story, 66 *B. anthracis*-positive samples were collected: 35 from desks, computers and keyboards, file cabinets, and mail slots. Spores were also found in 31 vacuum samples from the floor

Location	FBI (microbial forensic)	CDC (public health) and EPA (characterization)
Result	The FBI analysis of contamination patterns demonstrated that only one of three powders described by witnesses that had been received in AMI mail contained *B. anthracis* spores and that the attack letter was opened at the desk of an employee in the southwest corner of the first floor. Heavily contaminated items were removed for forensic comparisons	CDC epidemiologic and EPA environmental investigations determined the source of the patient's *B. anthracis* exposure to have been in the AMI building, as opposed to other locations such as his home. The extent of contamination was also determined by EPA
Postal mailboxes, N.J.		
Objective	To identify the mailbox from which the letters were mailed	Information not sought
Analysis	Because the four *B. anthracis*-contaminated envelopes recovered from Capitol Hill, the *New York Post*, and NBC were postmarked in Trenton, N.J., the FBI swabbed for *B. anthracis* hundreds of mailboxes, using traditional sampling methods, whose mail the Trenton mail processing facility had handled; the FBI developed an extender swab to sample some of these mailboxes	
Result	That letters, mailed from a heavily contaminated blue street box across the street from Princeton University's main entrance, were used as evidence supporting the FBI's conclusion that the perpetrator was a U.S. army scientist	
Congressional mailbag sampling, Washington, D.C. [b]		
Objective	To identify contaminated letters beyond what was discovered in Senator Daschle's office	Information not sought
Analysis	The FBI collected and quarantined more than 600 plastic bags of mail from all congressional buildings in a microbiological sampling approach that modified its existing collection, preparation, and analytic sampling processes. By assessing the level of spores in the mail bags with swab and air sampling, the FBI determined that one bag was more heavily contaminated than the others. Swab sampling identified 20 bags for manual and visual examination. Air sampling within those 20 bags then indicated that one bag was orders of magnitude more contaminated than all the others Rather than transport the samples to a laboratory for analysis, hazmat personnel directly inoculated culture media in the hazardous work area. [c]	

Location	FBI (microbial forensic)	CDC (public health) and EPA (characterization)
Result	Use of this approach led to the finding of the letter addressed to Senator Patrick Leahy that was heavily contaminated with dried *B. anthracis* spores. Tracking data indicated that this and other heavily contaminated envelopes had been processed through the same postal mail sorting equipment as, and within seconds, of two intentionally contaminated letters. This step was necessary to obtain information on how many letters were involved in the attack and their intended recipients, among other things. Evidence from this sampling also provided support for FBI's conclusions in its investigation	

Sources: (1) U.S. Department of Justice, *Amerithrax Investigative Summary* (Washington, D.C.: Feb. 19, 2010); (2) Douglas J. Beecher, "Forensic Application of Microbiological Culture Analysis to Identify Mail Intentionally Contaminated with *Bacillus anthracis* Spores," *Applied and Environmental Microbiology* 72 8 (Aug. 2006): 5304–10; (3) Lawrence Berkeley National Laboratory report.

[a]The AMI building is where the first victim worked.

[b]The FBI was already aware from its own investigation and the public health investigation that unopened spore-filled letters had released a sufficient number of spores to cause anthrax disease as well as extensive contamination at large postal facilities. It therefore concluded there should be enormous numbers of spores in congressional mailbags and that they should be easily identifiable by culture analysis.

[c]The FBI chose this approach because it stated it would be easier than using other analytic methods that required multiple steps to prepare samples as well as extensively trained technicians.

However, in its investigation, the FBI used additional methods beyond those it used for environmental sampling to further characterize the material in the envelopes, which in turn helped link the material to a source. For example, the FBI used scanning electron microscopy to obtain detailed information on spore characteristics.[6] Nevertheless, the FBI continues to rely on the methods public health authorities use when it samples indoor environments. For example, FBI officials also told us that the FBI now works with agencies such as CDC and EPA in responses involving environmental sampling. In a future bioterrorism incident, the FBI's sampling is likely to be simultaneous with or to follow initial sampling or environmental characterization. CDC and EPA have stated

[6]The methods, according to the FBI, included scanning electron microscopy, transmission electron microscopy, light microscopy, and high resolution SEM/energy-dispersive X-ray microanalysis to identify spore size, shape, and quality and the spatial profile of elements within the spore; inductively coupled plasma–optical emission spectroscopy to provide information regarding the elemental composition of the anthrax spore powders from the letters; gas chromatography mass spectrometry to characterize the anthrax spore powders with regard to the presence of agar (a growth medium); and accelerator mass spectrometry to identify the relative age of the material using 12 14 cc isotope ratios.

GAO-12-488 Anthrax Detection

that the FBI has its own methods and does not typically use the ones that
CDC developed through the LRN, and that while the devices may be
similar, they are not exactly the same. The environmental sampling
methods FBI used in its investigation of the 2001 *B. anthracis* release
were not validated.

Since the FBI's mission is not environmental monitoring, VSPWG
member agencies that perform environmental sampling take the lead in
development and validation of methods for environmental sample
collection. However, the FBI benefits from these efforts." For example, an
FBI official told us that the FBI has done side-by-side comparisons of
methods, including those of the LRN, which if they prove superior, could
be adapted for the FBI. It noted that it also has access to methods other
than those developed by the LRN. The FBI does not typically use the
LRN's sampling methods and validating its methods is outside the scope
of the DHS-led workgroup. DHS has established the NBFAC to address
the FBI's requirements for validating the methods it uses. NBFAC
currently has several ISO 17025 accredited analysis methods for
identifying and characterizing *B. anthracis*. Nevertheless, improvements
in sample collection procedures for the swab and wipe could be useful to
the FBI in developing its sampling plans or in evaluating its sampling
methods.

Appendix VI: Studies of Environmental Sampling Methods

Some of the studies DHS VSPWG agencies and others conducted to support the validation project are published in peer reviewed journals. These include CDC studies on the swab and wipe methods and a PNNL and SNL study on the performance gaps that were identified for the environmental sampling methods, such as the study addressing those gaps for the CDC cellulose sponge wipe method. EPA also conducted a study on its rapid-viability PCR method.

P. A. Krauter and others, "False Negative Rate and Other Performance Measures of a Sponge-Wipe Surface Sampling Method for Low Contaminant Concentrations," Applied and Environmental Microbiology 78(3) (December 2011): 846-54.

Paula A. Krauter and others, False Negative Rate and Other Performance Measures of a Sponge-Wipe Surface Sampling Method for Low Contaminant Concentrations, SAND2011-3395 (Albuquerque: Sandia National Laboratories, May 12, 2011).

G. F. Piepel and others, Experimental Design for a Sponge-Wipe Study to Relate the Recovery Efficiency and False Negative Rate to the Concentration of a Bacillus anthracis Surrogate for Six Surface Materials, PNNL-20060, Rev. 1, Pacific Northwest National Laboratory (Richland, Wash.: May 2011).

G. F. Piepel and others, Laboratory Studies on Surface Sampling of Bacillus anthracis Contamination: Summary, Gaps, and Recommendations, PNNL-20910 (Richland, Wash: Pacific Northwest National Laboratory, May 2011).

EPA also conducted a study and published a verification report on the rapid-viability PCR method.

S. E. Letant and others, "Rapid-Viability PCR Method for Detection of Live, Virulent Bacillus anthracis in Environmental Samples," Applied and Environmental Microbiology (September 2011): 6570–78.

EPA, Development and Verification of Rapid Viability Polymerase Chain Reaction (RV-PCR) Protocols for Bacillus Anthracis—For Application to Air Filters, Water and Surface Samples, EPA/600/R-10/156 (Livermore, Calif.: January 2011).

CDC's two-phase national validation study of the macrofoam swab method found in phase 1 (without dust) that premoistened macrofoam swabs recovered

- 25.7 percent (SD 15.2), 15.8 percent (SD 6.6), and 31.0 percent (10.9) for 101 and 102 and 104 spores per 26 cm2, respectively, of the spores from a nonporous surface where no dust was present, and

- in phase 2 of the study (with dust), using the protocol, swabs recovered

- 55.0 percent (SD 27.6), 27.9 percent (SD 15.9), and 42.0 percent (SD 25.0) for 101, 102, and 104 spores per 26 cm2, respectively, of spores when background dust was present.

    L. R. Hodges, L. J. Rose, H. O'Connell, and M. J. Arduino, "National Validation Study of a Swab Protocol for the Recovery of Bacillus anthracis *Spores from Surfaces,"* Journal of Microbiological Methods *81 (March 2010): 141–46.*

The percentage recovery was calculated as the number of spores recovered relative to the number of spores inoculated onto a steel surface or directly onto a swab (for positive controls), as determined by the analysis methods—culture and number of colony forming units (CFU).

A 2004 CDC study had already evaluated four swab materials (cotton, macrofoam, polyester, and rayon) and methods of processing to determine optimal *B. anthracis* spore recovery from steel surfaces, using *B. anthracis* Sterne.

    Laura Rose and others, "Swab Materials and Bacillus anthracis *Spore Recovery from Nonporous Surfaces,"* Emerging Infectious Diseases *10 (6) (June 2004): 1023–29.*

The study evaluated three methods of processing to remove spores from the swabs—vortexing, sonication, and minimal agitation. It also evaluated two swab preparations—premoistened and dry. It demonstrated that premoistened cotton and macrofoam swabs that were vortexed during processing were the most efficient (43.6 percent, SD of 11.1 percent, and 41.7 percent, SD 14.6 percent, respectively) while vortexed polyester and rayon were the least efficient (mean recovery of 9.9 percent, SD of 3.8 percent, and 11.5 percent, SD of 7.9 percent, respectively). It found that vortexing swabs for 2 minutes was superior to sonicating them for 12 minutes or using minimal agitation.

A 2006 CDC study evaluated a premoistened macrofoam swab processed by vortexing to recover *B. anthracis* Sterne spores from a steel surface. The swabs recovered 31.7 percent to 49.1 percent of spores from a ≤32.7 percent coefficient of variation in sampling precision and reproducibility for inocula of ≥38 spores.

L. R. Hodges and others, "Evaluation of a Macrofoam Swab Protocol for the Recovery of Bacillus anthracis *Spores from a Steel Surface," Applied and Environmental Microbiology (June 2006): 4429–30.*

Thus, CDC's 2010 national validation study (referenced above) included these two methods—macrofoam swab and vortexing. The study evaluated various performance parameters under low, medium, and high levels of spore contamination. For example, in phase 1, the performance of the swab at low concentrations (sampled swabs, spores only, with no dust added) was based on the direct inoculation of 49 spores onto a steel surface (SD of 7) and the inoculation of the control swabs with 42 spores (SD of 10), with sensitivities of 98.3 percent and 100 percent, respectively.[1]

The sensitivity of the method for both experimental phases was 98.3 percent for sampled swabs. Also, the addition of real-time (PCR) testing to the assay increased specificity from greater than 85.4 percent in phase 1 of the study to greater than 95 percent in phase 2. Although the precision was low at the 1 $\log 10$ inoculum level in both phases (56.9 percent and 40.0 percent), the swab processing protocol was sensitive, specific, precise, and reproducible at 2–4 $\log 10/26$ cm2 spore concentrations, according to the study.

In a 2011 CDC validation study of a cellulose sponge-wipe processing protocol for recovering, detecting, and quantifying viable *B. anthracis* Sterne spores from steel surfaces, steel coupons (645.16 cm3) were inoculated with 1-to 4-log(10) spores and then sampled with cellulose sponges (3M™ Sponge-Stick, St. Paul, Minnesota).

L. Rose and others, "National Validation Study of a Cellulose Sponge-Wipe Processing Method for Use After Sampling Bacillus anthracis *Spores from Surfaces," Applied and Environmental Microbiology (December 2011): 835–59*

The wipe is intended to be an alternative to the swab method, which is used for sampling small surface areas. The study noted that swabbing surfaces larger than 25.8 cm2 may reduce recovery efficiency.

---

[1]Direct inoculation refers to spreading the prepared spore suspension (inoculum) directly onto the swabs rather than on the steel coupons, which were then sampled with wipes. CDC personnel inoculated steel coupons measuring 26cm^2 1-4 log.

Surrogate dust and background organisms were added to the sponges to mimic environmental conditions. LRN-affiliated laboratories processed the sponges according to the protocol provided. Sensitivity, specificity, and mean percentage recovery between-laboratory (reproducibility), within-laboratory (precision), and total variance were calculated. The mean percentage recovery of spores (standard error) from the surface was 32.4 (4.4), 24.4 (2.8), and 30.1 (2.3) for 1-, 2-, and 4-log10 inoculum levels, respectively. Sensitivities for colony counts (as confirmed by PCR) were 84.1 percent, 100 percent, and 100 percent for 1-, 2-, and 4-log10 inocula, respectively. These data, according to the study, help characterize the variability of the processing method and thereby enhance confidence in the interpretation of the results of environmental sampling during a *B. anthracis* contamination investigation.

Regarding storing and shipping samples, a CDC study evaluated the viability of *B. anthracis* spores inoculated onto pre-moistened macrofoam swabs and stored at -15°, 5°, 21° and 35°C. Swabs were processed according to LRN culture protocols at 1, 2, 4 and 7 days, and the change in log10 recovery, as well as percent recovery, was calculated relative to day 0. Comparisons were made between recovery, with and without background dust and organisms, and between swabs packaged in primary containment only (transport bag) and swabs packaged in primary and secondary containment (transport bag placed into a 10-liter tinplate drum).

Swabs without background dust varied in spore recovery by ± 0.80 log10 of the day 0 recovery, and swabs with background dust varied by ± 0.014 log10 of the day 0 recovery, regardless of the storage temperature. Swabs stored at 5°C provided the most consistent spore recovery over all storage times. Swabs stored in both primary and secondary containment had less variability in spore recovery than if stored in primary containment alone, regardless of the storage time or temperature.

The presence of dust did not reduce the ability to recover *B. anthracis* spores, although if swabs were stored at 20° or 35°C for 48 hours or more, the background organisms in the dust multiplied, making it more difficult to identify *B. anthracis* in culture. Confirmation of colonies with PCR, however, demonstrated that positive identification was still possible ≥ 96 percent and 100 percent of the time at 102 and 104 spores per swab, respectively.

A. Perry, H. O'Connell, L. Rose, and J. Noble-Wang, *Storage Effects on Sample Integrity of Environmental Surface Sampling Specimens with Bacillus anthracis, Primary and Secondary Containment Spores.* Poster presented at the American Society for Microbiology Biodefense Conference, New Orleans, Louisiana, February 2, 2011.

Summary Report - A Perry and others. Storage Effects on Sample Integrity of Environmental Surface Sampling Specimens with *Bacillus anthracis* Spores. DHS IAA#HSHQDC-07-X00590 (February 2, 2011).

Finally, EPA developed and verified the rapid-viability PCR method for detection of live, virulent *B. anthracis* spores in wipe, air, and water samples. It published a study and a report on the method (both referenced above).

Criteria for assessing the method included methodology, limits of detection, accuracy with plating, absence of PCR and growth inhibition, and turnaround time for results, according to the verification report. Single laboratory verification of both manual and semi-automated versions of this optimized method showed limits of detection at the level of 10-spore-level (10-99 spores) per sample, both with and without debris, for all three sample types (clean laboratory water samples had a volume of 20 mL, wipes were 2-inch' squares of rayon-polyester gauze, and air filters were 47 mm diameter discs of hydrophobic polytetrafluoroethylene membranes).

Live *B. anthracis* Ames spores were consistently detected at the 10 spore level for both manual and semi-automated methods in heat-killed *B. anthracis* spore backgrounds of 106 colony-forming units per sample and combined nontarget backgrounds of 103 live *B. atrophaeus* subspecies *globigii* and 106 live *Pseudomonas aeruginosa.*

EPA officials stated in March 2012 that EPA anticipates a logical path of multi-laboratory validation of rapid-viability PCR method with selected sample types and a publication, but it will depend on the availability of funding.

Appendix VII: Interagency Validation Project Funding, Fiscal Years 2005–13

Validation of the methods for sample collection, transport, preparation, and analysis will be completed as funds, personnel resources, and competing priorities permit, according to DHS. Total funding obligated or planned for VSPWG activities from fiscal year 2005–13 was estimated at $16.3 million in February 2011. Funding for fiscal years 2005–11 was about $11.6 million of this amount. Estimated funding for fiscal years 2012–13 is about $4.7 million and is subject to availability. Of the project's total $16.3 million, each activity's total ranges from $100,000, for sample integrity studies, to about $5.6 million, for collection and analysis method studies. The collection and analysis methods (34 percent), field experiments (22 percent), and performance gap studies (16 percent) constitute the largest percentages of funding. Smaller percentages include validation of the VSP model at about 7 percent and confidence determination and statistical methods development at about 9 percent. External independent review and overall process validation is projected to be about 9 percent (fig. 6).

Figure 6: Validation Activities by Percentage of Total Project Funding, Fiscal Years 2005–13

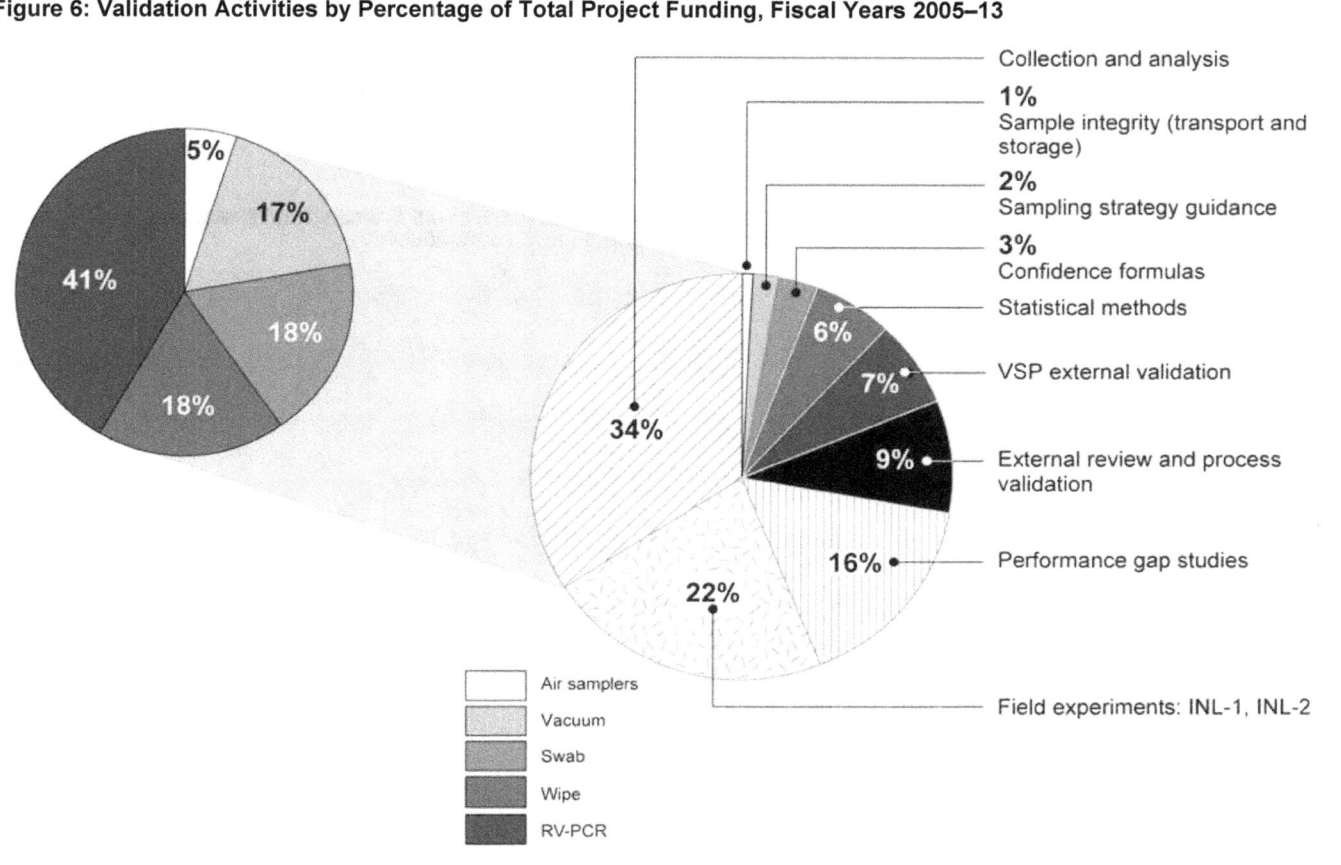

Source: GAO analysis of DHS 2011 data.

Note: N = $16,319,000 (100 percent).

Of the total $5.6 million (34 percent) for collection and analysis, the largest percentage is for developing, verifying, and evaluating the Rapid-Viability PCR method with selected sample types, at 41 percent, followed by the swab (18 percent), wipe (18 percent), and vacuum methods (17 percent). Efforts aimed at developing a probability-based sampling approach are covered under several activities in the roadmap, such as the performance gap studies, statistical methods, and external validation of the VSP model.[1]

Figure 7 breaks down the validation project's funding by fiscal year over its life, from fiscal year 2005 through funding projected for fiscal years 2012 and 2013.

Figure 7: Validation Funding, Fiscal Years 2005–13

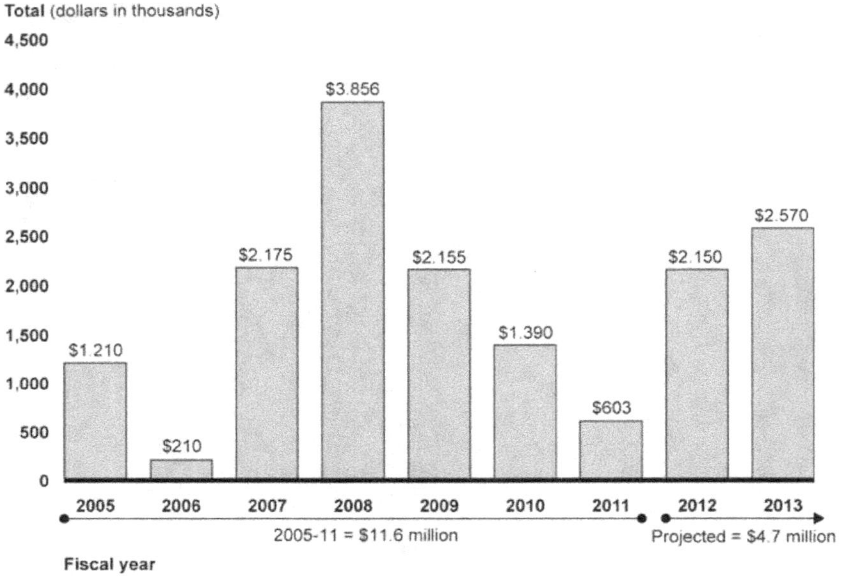

Total (dollars in thousands)

Fiscal year

Source: GAO analysis of DHS 2011data

- Fiscal year 2008 funding constituted the largest proportion of the total $16.3 million ($3.9 million or 24 percent). In that year, the second building experiment at INL was conducted, and EPA had begun research on developing and optimizing the Rapid viability PCR method for the Ames strain of *B. anthracis*, according to EPA. Each agency allocated funds in different amounts.

---

[1]Of the total $5.6 million, EPA provided about $2.6 million for its evaluation of the rapid-viability PCR method; CDC provided about $1,680,000 for its studies on the macrofoam swab and cellulose wipe methods, and it also projected $750,000 for its evaluation of the vacuum, for a total of about $2.4 million. DOD provided $600,000 for studies conducted by the Johns Hopkins Applied Physics laboratory on collection methods.

- Funding in fiscal year 2011 was the lowest ($603,000), other than fiscal years 2005 and 2006. Fiscal years 2005–06 were occupied in developing the strategic plan and deciding on a definition of validation. However, the first building experiment (INL-1) was conducted in fiscal year 2007, with funds allocated in fiscal year 2005 ($1 million) accounting for the majority of fiscal year 2005 funds.

- Projected funding for fiscal year 2013 is $2.6 million. Projected activities in fiscal years 2012–13 will primarily involve (1) CDC's studies for evaluating vacuum methods, (2) the performance gap studies at SNL, (3) PNNL's confidence determination and statistical methods development and external validation of the VSP model, and (4) external review and process validation.[2]

CDC and EPA have had a significant role in the VSPWG validation activities. They are involved in validating collection and analysis methods; have participated in the field experiments, including experiments involving probability sampling; and have been developing the sampling strategy guidance document. DOD actively participated in the building experiments at INL. NIST worked with PNNL in reviewing past chamber studies on the methods; and NIST, PNNL, and SNL worked on the performance gap studies. PNNL also developed the VSP model, advised VSPWG on validation issues, and provided input on the guidance document. By agency, funding obligated or estimated for CDC, DHS, DOD, and EPA totals about $2.8 million, $10 million, $775,000, and $2.8 million, respectively, for fiscal years 2005–13. Of the projected $4.7 million for fiscal years 2012-13, DHS is providing $3.9 million, and CDC is providing $750,000 for its evaluation of the vacuum. DHS will have provided the bulk of the funds for the VSPWG activities, at about $10 million, over the entire period, assuming projected funding becomes available.

---

[2]Projected funding for fiscal years 2012–13 depends on the availability of funds. Funding identified for sampling activities in conjunction with efforts of a broader scope, such as the INL building experiments are estimated components of the overall larger effort. PNNL funding may represent a component of a larger effort. Funding data do not necessarily match the activities listed in the roadmaps.

Completing all validation activities is scheduled for the end of fiscal year 2013. DHS acknowledged in July 2011 that it was difficult to say whether funds would be available to complete these activities, noting that the validation project has lower agency priority. A DHS official told us that it has been a challenge to get funding estimates from VSPWG's agencies and that the estimates it has obtained are imprecise.

Appendix VIII: Performance Parameters

The United States Pharmacopeia, ch. 1225, among others, describes performance parameters in detail:[1]

Accuracy

The accuracy of an analytical method is the closeness of test results obtained by that method to the true value. The accuracy of an analytical method should be established across its range.

False negative

Sample contains the analyte but tests negative. Finding of no contamination when in fact there is contamination.

False positive

Sample does not contain the analyte but tests positive. Finding of contamination when in fact there is no contamination.

Intermediate precision

Within-laboratories variations: different days, different analysts, different equipment, etc. Reproducibility expresses the precision between laboratories.

Limit of detection

The lowest amount of what is being analyzed (analyte) in a sample that can be detected, but not necessarily quantitated, under the stated experimental conditions. Limit tests substantiate that the amount of analyte is above or below a certain level. The detection limit is usually expressed as the concentration of analyte (e.g., percentage, parts per billion) in the sample.

Limit of quantitation

The lowest amount of analyte in a sample that can be determined with acceptable precision and accuracy under the stated experimental conditions. The quantitation limit is expressed as the concentration of analyte (e.g., percentage, parts per billion) in the sample.

---

[1]U.S. Pharmacopeia Convention, *United States Pharmacopeia*, ch. 1225, "Validation of Compendial Methods" (Rockville, Md.: United States Pharmacopeial, 2000), www.pharmacopeia.cn/v29240/usp29nf24s0_c1225.html.

Linearity

Ability of an analytical method to elicit test results that are directly, or by a well-defined mathematical transformation, proportional to the concentration of analyte in samples within a given range.

Precision

Precision may be a measure of either the degree of reproducibility or repeatability of the analytical method under normal operating conditions. The precision of an analytical method is the degree of agreement among individual test results when the method is applied repeatedly to multiple samplings of a homogeneous sample. The precision of an analytical method is usually expressed as the standard deviation or relative standard deviation (coefficient of variation) of a series of measurements.

Range

Interval between the upper and lower levels of analyte (including these levels) that has been demonstrated to be determined with a suitable level of precision, accuracy, and linearity using the method as written. The range for an analytical method is normally expressed in the same units as test results (e.g., percent, parts per million) obtained by the analytical method.

Repeatability

Use of the analytical procedure within a laboratory over a short period of time using the same analyst with the same equipment.

Reproducibility

The use of an analytical procedure in different laboratories, as in a collaborative study.

Robustness

A measure of the capacity of the method to remain unaffected by small but deliberate variations in the method parameters; provides a measure of reliability during normal use.

Ruggedness

Degree of reproducibility of test results obtained by the analysis of the same samples under a variety of conditions, such as different laboratories, analysts, instruments, lots of reagents, elapsed assay times, assay temperatures, or days. Ruggedness is normally expressed as the lack of influence on test results of operational and environmental variables of the analytical method. Ruggedness is a measure of reproducibility of test results under the variation in conditions normally expected from laboratory to laboratory and from analyst to analyst.

Sensitivity

The lowest and highest concentration of an analyte in a sample that can be quantitatively determined with an acceptable limit of precision and accuracy.

Specificity–selectivity

Ability to assess unequivocally the analyte in the presence of components that may be expected to be present, such as impurities, degradation products, and matrix components.

Appendix IX: Comments from the Department of Homeland Security

U.S. Department of Homeland Security
Washington, D.C. 20528

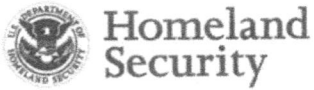

Homeland Security

June 4, 2012

Timothy M. Persons, Ph.D.
Chief Scientist
U.S. Government Accountability Office
441 G Street, NW
Washington, DC 20548

Ronald S. Fecso
Chief Statistician
U.S. Government Accountability Office
441 G Street, NW
Washington, DC 20548

Re: Draft Report GAO-12-488, "ANTHRAX: DHS Faces Challenges in Validating Methods for Sample Collection and Analysis"

Dear Dr. Persons and Mr. Fecso:

Thank you for the opportunity to review and comment on this draft report. The U.S. Department of Homeland Security (DHS) appreciates the U.S. Government Accountability Office's (GAO's) work in planning and conducting its review and issuing this report.

The Department is pleased to note GAO's positive recognition that DHS's Science and Technology Directorate working with other federal agencies, has made progress in addressing prior GAO recommendations regarding sampling methods for detecting *Bacillus anthracis* spores. For example, GAO acknowledged that the DHS-led working group has taken multiple actions to validate public health sampling methods (collection, transportation, extraction, analysis) and develop a statistical model that provides confidence statements when testing results are negative.

The draft report contained three recommendations designed to ensure that federal agencies have validated sampling methods for detecting *Bacillus anthracis* in indoor environments. Two recommendations were addressed to the Secretary of Homeland Security and one to the Secretary of Health and Human Services (HHS) and the Administrator of the Environmental Protection Agency (EPA). Regarding DHS, GAO recommended that the Secretary of Homeland Security:

Recommendation 1: Update the strategic plan and roadmap with an agreed-on scope and revised timelines.

Response: Concur. The Validated Sampling Plan Work Group led by DHS developed a consensus roadmap in August 2011, which will be revised to reflect appropriate scope and as well as to recognize subsequently delayed milestones caused by funding decrements to agency programs. Additionally, it is DHS's intention to update the strategic plan to reflect the advances made by the group since 2007 and the remaining tasks to be addressed in achieving the goals participating agencies jointly agreed to and outlined in the 2006 Memorandum of Understanding (MOU). We note, however, that the support of HHS and EPA will be essential to completing this update.

Recommendation 2: Complete the validation project, including validating the collection methods and completing related ongoing studies.

Response: Concur. DHS intends to fulfill its obligations as described in the 2006 MOU. DHS believes that Incident Commanders should have well-founded options for conducting sampling campaigns in contaminated structures and appreciates GAO recognition of efforts to outline and characterize those options.

Again, thank you for the opportunity to review and comment on this draft report. Technical comments for the report were previously provided under separate cover. Please feel free to contact me if you have any questions. We look forward to working with you on future Homeland Security issues.

Sincerely,

Jim H. Crumpacker
Director
Departmental GAO-OIG Liaison Office

2

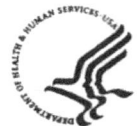

DEPARTMENT OF HEALTH & HUMAN SERVICES

OFFICE OF THE SECRETARY

Assistant Secretary for Legislation
Washington, DC 20201

JUN 19 2012

Timothy M. Persons, Ph.D.
Chief Scientist
U.S. Government Accountability Office
441 G Street NW
Washington, DC 20548

Dear Mr. Persons:

Attached are comments on the U.S. Government Accountability Office's (GAO) report entitled:
"Anthrax: DHS Faces Challenges in Validating Methods for Sample Collection and Analysis"
(GAO-12-488).

The Department appreciates the opportunity to review this draft section of the report prior to
publication.

Sincerely,

Jim R. Esquea
Assistant Secretary for Legislation

Attachment

cc: Ron Fecso, Chief Statistician

<u>**GENERAL COMMENTS OF THE DEPARTMENT OF HEALTH AND HUMAN
SERVICES (HHS) ON THE GOVERNMENT ACCOUNTABILITY OFFICE'S (GAO)
DRAFT REPORT ENTITLED, "ANTHRAX: DHS FACES CHALLENGES IN
VALIDATING METHODS FOR SAMPLE COLLECTION AND ANALYSIS" (GAO-12-
488)**</u>

Background

The Department appreciates the opportunity to comment on this draft report.

GAO Report Recommendations

The Department of Homeland Security (DHS) should

- *Update the strategic plan and roadmap with an agreed-on scope and revised timelines.*
- *Complete the validation project, including validating the collection methods in a laboratory setting, in a manner that determines the potential sources of variation in collection method performance, including variation that could be introduced by individual samplers.*
- *Complete related ongoing studies.*

We also recommend that the HHS Secretary and the Administrator of the Environmental Protection Agency (EPA) support DHS in its goal of achieving (1) validated sampling methods to understand the limitations of the data that would be provided to decision makers, and (2) a mutually acceptable, statistically based sampling approach that can be employed in those situations in which decision makers—such as incident commanders and others—conclude that statistical confidence statements need to be made about the level of contamination in a particular indoor environment.

HHS agrees that additional work needs to be done to address gaps in anthrax sampling strategies and methods for deriving confidence limits around the results, and is supportive of the recommendation that DHS (in consultation with HHS and EPA) should update the strategic plan and roadmap with an agreed upon scope and timeline.

HHS does not agree with the remaining GAO recommendations, but suggests that DHS (in consultation with HHS and EPA) should:

- Complete related ongoing studies, including evaluating collection methods in a laboratory setting, in order to gain better estimates of variation in the steps in the process; and
- For scientifically defensible sampling approaches, pursue the development of confidence statements about the level of contamination in a particular indoor environment under those situations in which decision makers—such as incident commanders and others—conclude that it is needed (e.g., when initial results are all non-detect).

Much of the discussion of this report among experts has centered on targeted sampling approaches versus a statistically based sampling approach. Because of the almost limitless

1

GENERAL COMMENTS OF THE DEPARTMENT OF HEALTH AND HUMAN
SERVICES (HHS) ON THE GOVERNMENT ACCOUNTABILITY OFFICE'S (GAO)
DRAFT REPORT ENTITLED, "ANTHRAX: DHS FACES CHALLENGES IN
VALIDATING METHODS FOR SAMPLE COLLECTION AND ANALYSIS" (GAO-12-
488)

number of variables from one environmental contamination event to the next, a statistically
based sample approach is not generally going to be feasible. The sampling methodology
employed should be determined by the nature of the event, the environmental complexities, and
the actions that may occur based on the testing results. No matter the sampling approach, HHS
believes emphasis should be placed on understanding, and to the extent possible, defining the
confidence in the contamination estimates and the limitations of the analyses.

Below are some general HHS comments that address concerns about technical aspects pertinent
to GAO's recommendations:

Validated Sampling Methods

GAO recommends that HHS support DHS in achieving validated sampling methods for detecting
B. anthracis in potentially contaminated areas. GAO has concerns that existing methods may not
be sufficient to detect low levels of contamination in field situations.

HHS acknowledges that laboratory validation is very important. During anthrax investigations,
the CDC's Laboratory Response Network (LRN)[1] uses fully validated laboratory-analytical
methods to confirm the presence of *B. anthracis*. However, HHS notes that field settings are less
controlled than laboratory settings. For this reason, it is HHS's position that there are
insurmountable challenges to applying similar standards to field settings and that any attempt to
do so would result in data that would not be applicable to an actual event.

Regarding GAO's recommendation regarding determination of the variation attributable to
multiple samplers, HHS believes that reducing and defining individual variation in collection
methods is better approached through training, in post-training evaluation, and during
competency assessments under simulated field conditions in a laboratory setting.

The need for further extensive validation of currently employed sampling methods may be
limited to completing current studies and closing any newly identified gaps. CDC already has
fully validated swab and wipe processing and analysis methods for detecting *B. antracis* in a
laboratory setting, which is consistent with the definition of validation under the International
Standard (ISO 17025). CDC is focusing its efforts on evaluating several differently vacuum
sampling methods to identify a suitable method for future laboratory validation work involving
porous surfaces.

---

[1] Laboratory Response Network - a national network of local, state, and federal public health, food testing,
veterinary diagnostic, and environmental testing laboratories that provide the laboratory infrastructure and capacity
to respond to biological and chemical terrorism, and other public health emergencies. The more than 150
laboratories that make up the LRN are affiliated with federal agencies, military installations, international partners,
and state/local public health departments.

2

**GENERAL COMMENTS OF THE DEPARTMENT OF HEALTH AND HUMAN
SERVICES (HHS) ON THE GOVERNMENT ACCOUNTABILITY OFFICE'S (GAO)
DRAFT REPORT ENTITLED, "ANTHRAX: DHS FACES CHALLENGES IN
VALIDATING METHODS FOR SAMPLE COLLECTION AND ANALYSIS" (GAO-12-
488)**

Statistically Based Sampling Approach

GAO recommends that HHS support DHS in developing a statistically based sampling approach
for use in a field setting because GAO believes that statistical sampling will give decision
makers more reliable information to determine whether or not a potentially contaminated
building is "safe." The statistical sampling approach requires the collection of random samples
to obtain a specified level of confidence that a high percentage of a building or area has no
detectable contamination. Statistical sampling requires the collection of a high number of
samples and therefore requires extensive human resources and equipment to rapidly process this
volume of samples. In contrast to the statistical sampling approach, the targeted sampling
approach, which is currently used, uses professional judgment and, when available,
epidemiologic information to select locations in the environment most likely to be contaminated.
This information is used to make decisions about the location and number of samples to be
collected as well as to inform environmental and public health action as the assessment of
contamination and decontamination processes are occurring.

HHS does not concur with GAO's recommendation, which implies a need for statistically based
sampling methods in field scenarios. What is needed are scientifically defensible sampling
approaches (e.g., targeted and statistical sampling approaches) that can inform incident
commanders and other decision makers with critical information, including limitations of the
procedures and estimates of confidence limits. The following statements support this
conclusion:

1. CDC has successfully used targeted sampling approaches to identify contamination in several
post-2001 anthrax events. For example, a targeted sampling approach was used in the 2009 New
Hampshire investigation that successfully identified low levels (close to the levels of detection of
contamination) in the building of concern.

2. Statistical sampling is labor and resource intensive, exhausting capacity and detracting from
the overall government response at times when rapid response is most critical. HHS has
concerns that applying this approach would dramatically impact response times and
inappropriately direct much-needed resources to collecting and processing more samples than are
required to adequately assess risk.

3. HHS notes that there are rare circumstances under which HHS/CDC would consider using a
statistical sampling approach during the initial response, but the use of statistical sampling is
limited by the following: (1) the availability of qualified staff, personal protective equipment,
and sampling supplies to conduct the sampling; and (2) the need to maintain situational
awareness as the event unfolds and maintain capacity to rapidly conduct targeted sampling at
other priority sites as they are identified. Underscoring recognition by HHS/CDC of the role for
statistical based sampling, CDC has a software module for statistically based sampling in the rare
circumstances where it is required. While this product could benefit from further refinement, it

3

GENERAL COMMENTS OF THE DEPARTMENT OF HEALTH AND HUMAN SERVICES (HHS) ON THE GOVERNMENT ACCOUNTABILITY OFFICE'S (GAO) DRAFT REPORT ENTITLED, "ANTHRAX: DHS FACES CHALLENGES IN VALIDATING METHODS FOR SAMPLE COLLECTION AND ANALYSIS" (GAO-12-488)

is functional for the limited public health needs. Further development of statistical approaches is not necessary.

Conclusion

HHS agrees that additional work should be done to address gaps in anthrax sampling strategies and methods for deriving confidence limits around the results. HHS is supportive of the recommendation that DHS (in consultation with HHS and EPA) should update the strategic plan and roadmap with an agreed upon scope and timeline. HHS does not agree with the remaining GAO recommendations, but suggests that:

DHS (in consultation with HHS and EPA) complete related ongoing studies, including evaluating collection methods in a laboratory setting, in order to gain better estimates of variation in the steps in the process; and for scientifically defensible sampling approaches, pursue the development of confidence statements about the level of contamination in a particular indoor environment under those situations in which decision makers—such as incident commanders and others—conclude that it is needed (e.g., when initial results are all non-detect).

4

Appendix XI: Comments from the Environmental Protection Agency

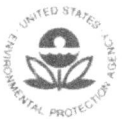

UNITED STATES ENVIRONMENTAL PROTECTION AGENCY
WASHINGTON, D.C. 20460

MAY 1 7 2012

OFFICE OF
SOLID WASTE AND
EMERGENCY RESPONSE

Dr. Timothy M. Persons, Ph.D.
Chief Scientist
Government Accountability Office
Washington, DC 20548

Dear Dr. Persons:

I am transmitting the Agency's response to the Government Accountability Office (GAO) April 30, 2012 report entitled "Anthrax – DHS Faces Challenges in Validating Methods for Sample Collection and Analysis. The Environmental Protection Agency (EPA) appreciates the opportunity to comment on the report. These comments reflect consolidated input from both the Office of Solid Waste and Emergency Response (OSWER) and the Office of Research and Development (ORD). The Agency is submitting overall and specific comments which have been shared with you previously during the drafting of the report, Agency interviews, and on the Statement of Facts.

GAO has still made the following recommendations in its latest report (1) update the strategic plan's and roadmap's scope and timelines, and (2) complete the validation project. It also stated that the Secretary of Health and Human Services (HHS) and the Administrator of the EPA should support completion of the Department of Homeland Security's (DHS) goal regarding the development of a mutually acceptable statistically based sampling approach.

We are concerned that GAO continues to not recognize that the overall response on Capitol Hill was successful using targeted sampling and studies such as at Idaho National Labs continue to re-enforce the effectiveness of targeted sampling. A statistically based approach is not needed from a science perspective and it is also not possible with today's realities. Moreover, the environmental laboratory analytical capacity that would be needed does not exist for a statistically based sampling approach, nor does the manpower to support sampling, and the software to handle the data is not available without significant cost investments. There are larger gaps that need to be filled to address bacillus anthracis decontamination.

EPA can participate with DHS in updating its strategic plan and in completing validation efforts as appropriate. However, EPA cannot agree to a statistically based sampling approach. As an alternate proposal, EPA recommends that it develop a policy paper that clearly explains how confidence statements can be made when using targeted sampling approaches, combined with additional sampling related information (e.g., weighting based upon incident specific information) and approaches (e.g., composite sampling methods or new, validated sampling methods). EPA can apply the results of the body of research that has been completed as well as professional operational experience to develop this paper and demonstrate that statistical based sampling approaches are not necessary to make confidence statements.

We look forward to implementing EPA's recommendation that we believe is consistent with the science or our experience in the field.

Sincerely,

Mathy Stanislaus
Assistant Administrator

Enclosure

2

Appendix XII: GAO Contacts and Staff Acknowledgments

GAO Contacts	Timothy M. Persons (Chief Scientist), (202) 512-6412 or personst@gao.gov.
Staff Acknowledgments	In addition to the contact named above, Sushil Sharma, Assistant Director; and James Ashley; Hazel Bailey; Justin Fisher; Mae Liles; Penny Pickett; and Elaine Vaurio made key contributions to this report.

Related GAO Products

Federal Agencies Have Taken Some Steps to Validate Sampling Methods and to Develop a Next-Generation Anthrax Vaccine, GAO-06-756T (Washington D.C.: May 9, 2006).

Anthrax Detection: Agencies Need to Validate Sampling Activities in Order to Increase Confidence in Negative Results, GAO-05-251 (Washington D.C.: March 31, 2005).

U.S. Postal Service: Better Guidance Is Needed to Ensure an Appropriate Response to Anthrax Contamination, GAO-04-239 (Washington D.C.: September 9, 2004).

U.S. Postal Service: Issues Associated with Anthrax Testing at the Wallingford Facility, GAO-03-787T (Washington D.C.: May 19, 2003).

U.S. Postal Service: Better Guidance Is Needed to Improve Communication Should Anthrax Contamination Occur in the Future, GAO-03-316 (Washington D.C.: April 7, 2003).

GAO's Mission	The Government Accountability Office, the audit, evaluation, and investigative arm of Congress, exists to support Congress in meeting its constitutional responsibilities and to help improve the performance and accountability of the federal government for the American people. GAO examines the use of public funds; evaluates federal programs and policies; and provides analyses, recommendations, and other assistance to help Congress make informed oversight, policy, and funding decisions. GAO's commitment to good government is reflected in its core values of accountability, integrity, and reliability.
Obtaining Copies of GAO Reports and Testimony	The fastest and easiest way to obtain copies of GAO documents at no cost is through GAO's website (www.gao.gov). Each weekday afternoon, GAO posts on its website newly released reports, testimony, and correspondence. To have GAO e-mail you a list of newly posted products, go to www.gao.gov and select "E-mail Updates."
Order by Phone	The price of each GAO publication reflects GAO's actual cost of production and distribution and depends on the number of pages in the publication and whether the publication is printed in color or black and white. Pricing and ordering information is posted on GAO's website, http://www.gao.gov/ordering.htm. Place orders by calling (202) 512-6000, toll free (866) 801-7077, or TDD (202) 512-2537. Orders may be paid for using American Express, Discover Card, MasterCard, Visa, check, or money order. Call for additional information.
Connect with GAO	Connect with GAO on Facebook, Flickr, Twitter, and YouTube. Subscribe to our RSS Feeds or E-mail Updates. Listen to our Podcasts. Visit GAO on the web at www.gao.gov.
To Report Fraud, Waste, and Abuse in Federal Programs	Contact: Website: www.gao.gov/fraudnet/fraudnet.htm E-mail: fraudnet@gao.gov Automated answering system: (800) 424-5454 or (202) 512-7470
Congressional Relations	Katherine Siggerud, Managing Director, siggerudk@gao.gov, (202) 512-4400, U.S. Government Accountability Office, 441 G Street NW, Room 7125, Washington, DC 20548
Public Affairs	Chuck Young, Managing Director, youngc1@gao.gov, (202) 512-4800 U.S. Government Accountability Office, 441 G Street NW, Room 7149 Washington, DC 20548